Israel:

The Start-up Nation for Medical Innovation

DR. ROB NORMAN

CONTENTS

ACKNOWLEDGMENTS

I have many people to thank for helping this book come to fruition. For those I have interviewed and have included in these pages, it certainly has been a true pleasure to listen and grow from your stories. I hope that I have succeeded in bringing your achievements to a wider audience. We live in a time of incredible growth and potential and I am happy to highlight a portion of the amazing accomplishments by the Israeli people. I am especially proud of my opportunity to serve the people of Israel through the Jewish National Fund and other volunteer groups.

Love to my family and friends, fellow physicians, students, office staff, and to all those that add a creative spark to the world and make it a better place in which to live.

My great appreciation goes to Jon Medved for his work around the world in support of Israel and innovation. Russell Robinson, Gideon Shavit, Uri Smajovits, Ken Segel, Rick Krosnick, Glen Schwartz, Dr.

Melinda Wolf, Sharon David, Ron Lauder, Beth Morris,
Rick Rappaport, Ida Rae Chernin, Tina Gordon, Mary
Ellen Hogan, and all members of the JNF Tampa Bay
Board of Directors, Cindy Spahn and all the Kosher
Hammies, Ron Kriss, Bruce Gould, Jeffrey Levine, Dr.
Sol Lizerbram, Dr. Ronna Schneider, Anne Tishkoff, Issy
Herzog, Sharad Paul, Marina Furman, Jessica Schapiro,
Talia Aviani, Dr. Fred Cohen, Dr. Avrum Pollock and all
JNF DFI members, Dan Berman, Yedidya Harush, Dr.
Vivien and Don Wong, Dr. Marissa Potter, Dick Greco,
Pam Iorio, Sandra Freedman, Rabbi Leor Sinai, Orit
Rome, Susan Turner, Linda Ruescher, Rabbi Yossi
Kahana, Elaine Viders, Bill Sefekar, Dr. Charlie and
Karen Vega, Mark Schlanger, Ida Rae Chernin, Laura
Salzer, Dr. Stu Lipman, Laurie and Marty Kleiner, Rande
Friedman, Dan Sultan, Ernie and Judy Lisi, Jeff Vinik,
Bob Buckhorn, Stephen Muss, Rabbi Lazer Rivkin, Erin
Abel, Rabbi Nathan Farb, Rabbi Richard Birnholz, Mayor
Ruvik Danilovich, Rabbi Zalman Blecher, Ed Shindle,
Dr. Rob Lewenson, Dr. Dennis Lewinson, Elizabeth
Gelman, Judy Genshaft, David Scher, Mark Wright, Dr.
Zena Lansky, Jack Ross, Dr. Barry Levine, Rabbi Levi
Rivkin, Rabbi Uriel Rivkin, Dr. Rick Miller, Dr. Richard

Brown, Dr. Lon Lynn, Dr. Ken Webster, Drs. Kiran and Pallavi Patel, Dr. Ken Forster, Dr. Harvey Feld, Dr. Mel Konner, Bob Warchola, Ron Fraley, Andrew Shein, Carole Fluhart, Dr. William Eng, Elaine Adler, Dr. Ben Barankin, Rita Rosenkranz, Dr. Brett Scotch, Dr. Carl Zeilonka, Dave and Candace Bowers, Eric Man, Arch Deal, Gary Gould, Mark Segel, Dr. Leonid Eidelman, Dr. Zeev Feldman, Lynn Lafferty, DL Xie, Marty Yost, Mike Sobel, Rabbi Mendy Dubrowski, Frank Delargy, Elise Cundiff, Sheldon Wolf, Denise Brown, Pam Liflander, Rick and Ellyne Myers, Andrea Graham, Steve Silverman, Janet and Eric Nichols, Mark Schlanger, Ambassador Gideon Meir and many others have all been loyal friends and advisors. Thanks much to Dr. Michele Melamed for a great introduction to the book and for helping me to organize interviews and chapters. I'm very proud of you and it has been a great privilege to teach you as a medical student and encourage you as an emergency medicine resident. Thanks to Ibsen Morales for all his hard work and support.

PREFACE

It is no exaggeration to say that healthcare is undergoing a revolution no less earth-shaking than the discovery of germ theory or the introduction of antibiotics. Digital health – the application of digital technologies to healthcare – is transforming our approach to medicine and improving our well-being. As the global population ages and healthcare demands accelerate, supplies and services cannot keep pace. Digital health solutions offer the promise of delivering more for less – and hold the potential to positively impact the lives of current and future generations.

Nowhere is this revolution more evident than in Israel, where 100% of the healthcare system is digitized, both at the individual patient level and throughout its organizations. As *The Lancet* observed, "With its many start-up enterprises, Israel encourages digital innovation and this culture will help tackle some of the key challenges facing the country's health systems." In fact, Israel-based companies are helping healthcare systems in other countries get online and get secure, efficient and cost-effective. The statistics are impressive:

There has been strong growth in the number of new digital health companies established in recent years, with 385 locally founded companies in 2016. These companies are an important part of a thriving life sciences startup industry that has had a major impact on the country's economy with more than USD 7.2 billion in multiple mergers and acquisitions in 2015, a sizeable increase from the preceding year. Israel was also an early adopter of digital health technologies in clinical practice, with big data analytics, telemedicine, and online patient engagement widely incorporated into daily clinical care.

The latest milestone was the launch of a space laboratory developed by Israel's SpacePharma, which arrived at the International Space Station in November 2017. This was the first time that a full lab system was launched to the ISS.

As a leading investor in medical technology, OurCrowd has worked diligently to recognize the potential of Israeli startups and bring them the capital and global growth network they need. A few examples from the portfolio gave an idea of how exciting we believe this field is:

- MedAware, which helps ensure patients get the right prescription, saving lives and potentially saving more than $13 billion annually in the U.S. alone

- Healthy.IO, which is turning smartphones into medical imaging tools for full-fledged diagnostics

- Zebra Medical Vision, which in November 2017 struck a deal with Google to use its AI algorithms, and also rolled out a new model offering $1 medical scans that can detect liver and lung disease

- DreaMed, whose groundbreaking cloud-based analytics and decision support technology act as an artificial pancreas to regulate insulin

OurCrowd unveiled the first digital health fund in Israel in late 2016, recognizing the sector as one of the fastest growing in terms of funding and M&A activity. The fund's exclusive focus is important given the complexity of healthcare delivery and markets.

OurCrowd is also a partner with Hebrew University, Israel's leading academic institution, to sponsor an MBA program for biomedical management. The program is the first of its kind in Israel, and aims to provide new top-notch talent for the forward-thinking market.

We are proud to be part of the medical innovation revolution that has so much potential to improve people's daily lives everywhere across the globe. I'm hopeful Dr. Norman's book will help bring this story of hope and achievement to a broad audience.

Jon Medved

Founder and CEO, OurCrowd

INTRODUCTION

Israel is a country where various religions, cultures, dialects, arts and history collide. Israel is a land where human beings, animals, and the test of "survival of the fittest" exist in its full capacity. Israel is one of the centers of the world for innovation, political and economic gains, and the opportunity for personal and professional growth beyond measure. And Israel is so small one has to squint to locate it on a map.

The State of Israel hasn't been around long, and the land before 1948 was left dry and barren from a hostile environment. The history of the Jewish people is filled with expulsion, persecution and desecration. With a lengthy exile of some two thousand years, the Jews were left to wander and resort to the one thing they knew best, prayer and faith. The connection to their creator, the Almighty, has served them well by nurturing and sustaining their unbounded love for the land of their forefathers. The Jews had trekked from ancient Egypt across a huge wasteland to Israel, which was essentially another poor area of desolation. The ability to use one's imagination for a future filled with richness and contentment was as important then as it is today.

If it wasn't for risk-taking individuals such as David Ben-Gurion, Golda Meir, Menachem Begin, Yitzchak Rabin, Shimon Peres, and others, who had extraordinary vision and tremendous courage to take steps on behalf of their people, Israel would not be in the position it is today. Though the Holocaust may have left us smaller in numbers, it did not diminish our fervent dream to become innovators for change, creativity and to contribute to the world.

And that's exactly what has happened. With the highest number of startups per capita in the world, it is no wonder why Israel has been labeled the "Start-Up Nation." Despite being attacked multiple times in major wars since its inception and in numerous other "smaller battles", Israel has overcome enormous adversity and has built incubators for success from the ground up. Growth doesn't happen automatically, and the combination of water, fertilizer, and back-breaking manual labor and ingenuity came together so that the trees, the land and the country's people grew against all odds. Agriculture becomes challenging with little water at one's disposal, but through technology such as drip irrigation, Israel has been able to yield high quality crops, clean water, and an overall water surplus.

The Israeli techniques have been copied by other countries around the world, particularly in certain areas of Asia and Africa lacking access to purified water and clean fruits and vegetables. Thousands of people from other countries come to Israel each year to train in the Central Arava and other agricultural areas to learn and import the Israeli techniques back to their homes. As the world's populations continue to boom, so does the need for cleaner environments and resources to recycle waste proficiently. Israel has taken on the critical role of constructing solar power generators and seawater detoxification systems. It has proved to other countries that its cutting-edge technology will drastically expand the health and living standards of millions of people worldwide.

Israel has been at the forefront of research and

development in many areas, particularly with the rise of technology and the seemingly irreplaceable computer. The original Intel 8088 processor was developed in Israel. More recently, the Kindle reader used by Amazon is successful today because of the technology created in Israel. Artificial intelligence, nanotechnology, medicine, and pharmacology are just some of the many disciplines where Israeli scientists are actively taking key roles in creating and developing new technologies.

Israeli physicians and engineers have tapped into the realm of neuroplasticity and discovered new brain functions and adaptations. Cancer treatments and other lifesaving devices have emerged from innovators and medical startups funded by the Israeli government.

The realized potential for human creativity and execution of ideas coming from Israel is truly remarkable. The path to greatness for this little country is filled with obstacles, but nothing really seems to deter its people from contributing to our new age of discovery.

Israel is committed to the construction of a better,

healthier and peaceful world. Prosperity and freedom are some of the virtues embedded in the foundation with which Israel was created. Though it remains a flashpoint of world controversy, constantly facing terrorism and the threat of war, it remains steadfast in its pursuits.

Since 1948, Israel has truly been a light unto the nations. Israelis depend on strong national leadership; its politicians are dedicated to ensuring that the education, intellectual pursuits, and improvement of health of its citizens take center stage. An essential ingredient to the success of Israel is that it has worked hard to establish an environment for creativity, with freedom to explore and take risks. Although it is a small country, with perhaps more media attention than any other nation in the world, Israel's desire for peace and the price it pays for that resolution is not often obvious. Despite the distorted view certain people have of Israel and its people, it continues to yearn for harmony, for growth, and for perpetual contributions to the world.

The collective responsibility in all acts of life along with individual ambition has helped breed the innovations described in this book you are about to read. Israel has created a society based upon meritocracy. Efforts in ingenuity are expected. From the creation of cherry tomatoes to lifesaving drugs and devices such as the Pill-Cam, Israelis take pride in their passion for technology. I hope you will enjoy every word forthcoming and that you will come away being more educated in the marvelous innovations coming out of Israel today. The world is changing rapidly, and Israel wants to remain the innovative powerhouse of the globe and always be ahead of the game. Just watch. You'll see and be amazed.

Dr. Michele Melamed

OVERVIEW

How is it that Israel, with just 8.5 million people, only 69 years old, with few natural resources and minimal infrastructure, is a world leader in producing medical and biotechnology start-ups and companies and is first in the world for medical device patents per capita? Israel is surrounded by enemies trying to wipe it out. The country has been in constant war and turmoil since its founding in 1948, yet thrives in adversity. Economies as diverse as Dubai, India, Ireland, and Singapore have tried to mimic the "Israel effect."

On my many trips to Israel as the national chairman of the Jewish National Fund's Doctors for Israel, I have observed the amazing life-saving and life-enhancing advances of Israeli medicine and discussed the future of medicine and science with many leading scientists. I visited the makers of ReWalk robotic exoskeleton (featured on the hit TV show "Glee") that enables paraplegic runners in London and Tel Aviv to complete marathons and spent time at Given Imaging's PillCam capsule endoscopy company. The list of amazing technologies provided by Israel keeps growing. I want to make this very clear--I am not just a medical and technical Zionist, but a supporter for all of Israel and its many and varied people.

Among the numerous people on the cutting edge of Israeli medicine and science is Eran Perry, managing director at Israel Health Care Ventures (IHCV), one of the largest venture capital funds in the country. "It's almost a cliché to say Israel is an excellent place for medical innovation," Perry said in an interview. "But if you look at global statistics, it's evident — from the total expenditure on civilian R&D, where we are ranked first; to human infrastructure and entrepreneurship, where we rank in the top five. You can see the results in patents. We are first in the world for medical device patents per capita, and second in Europe for bio-pharma."

I believe this is one of the most important times in the history of medicine and science and that Israel plays a key role. According to the newest data, more than 1,000 Israeli companies are in healthcare or life-science products, including 700 in medical devices, and approximately half are already generating revenue. I will highlight numerous accomplishments by Israeli medicine and science companies and provide compelling reasons why Israel is a world center in innovation.

My belief is the medical and science entrepreneurial spirit resides not just in Israel, but in Jews, and promotes an innovative culture. Not always satisfied with what the world currently offers (we like to kvetch), there is a drive to improve life and perform Tikkun Olam (repairing the world) whenever the opportunity arises, reflected in the numbers of Jews in medicine and the helping professions. At least 181 Jews and people of half- or three-quarters-Jewish ancestry have been awarded the Nobel Prize, and 22% of all individual recipients worldwide between 1901 and 2010 and 36% of all US recipients during the same period were Jewish. Of all organizations awarded the Nobel Peace Prize, 25% were founded principally by Jews or by people of half-Jewish descent. Not bad, considering Jews currently make up approximately 0.2% of the world's population. Of course, many Jews in national and local environments have also done their share. And many of our Moslem, Christian, Hindu, and other brothers and sisters in the world have helped create a wonderful mix of innovation and productivity in medicine and science.

For both medical and other small-to-medium-sized companies, acquisition is proving to be the sought-after path. In 2015, deals generated a total of $7.2 billion, compared to 2014 deals that yielded $5 billion. This 44 percent increase is primarily due to large multinational corporations' eager to acquire innovative technologies. In the last decade, there has been $21b invested in Israeli start-ups. Over the past six years there has been over 400 exits totaling over $20b. Rubi Suliman, high tech partner at PwC Israel, said in a statement that, "We have grown accustomed to the presence in Israel of global giants like Facebook, Apple, IBM, Qualcomm, Microsoft, Intel and more." Israel has more NASDAQ listed companies than any other country besides the US. Additionally, with 4500+ start-ups founded in the past five years alone, the greater Tel Aviv area is ranked #1 in the world for innovative capacity by the IMD Global Competitiveness Year Book.

During a recent trip to Israel with participants from our Jewish National Fund's Doctors for Israel group, we were provided with a two hour talk from Dr. Leonid Eidelman, the President of the Israeli Medical Association, and Dr. Zeev Feldman, the Chairman of the Israeli Medical Association World Fellowship, at the headquarters of the Israeli Medical Association The two explained in detail how they and their groups work to represent Israeli doctors and help to advance medical care and support practicing physicians across Israel. In addition, they spoke in detail about the unique relationships between Israel and doctors from around the world. Many Israeli doctors do specialty training and research in the United States and in other countries and many doctors from outside Israel do advanced work in Israel before returning to their own countries.

I have interviewed many of the key people in the world who are at the core of this exciting revolution in Israeli medicine and biotechnology. The answers as to Israel's success have been consistent and will be expanded on in each chapter. Along with one of the most educated and entrepreneurial populations in the world, Israel is an ideal birthplace of innovation. The Jewish tradition of questioning and open-minded exploration of seemingly impossible tasks has fueled the fire for Israel to become a world leader in medicine and innovation. Mandatory military service as a dynamic resource for character-building, extended social interactions and aggressive recruitment by start-ups, government policies that fund innovation, and the immigrant influx have all played vital roles in Israel's growth and are covered in detail. In addition, I have included extensive information based on interviews with those who do business with Israel, including those in the United States such as the Cleveland Clinic Global Healthcare Innovations Alliance, and many other leading entrepreneurs. The narrative is filled with colorful characters and often humorous tales; this book will inform, entertain, and hopefully leave you having a greater awareness of Israel and wanting to learn more.

New and innovative ideas in medicine and biotechnology sprout up daily in a robust fashion, despite all the hardships and limitations in Israel. Inside the covers of this book you will not only get a great feel for the amazing events happening now in Israel, but you will acquire wonderful, motivational and informative tips for your own life on how a never-say-never mentality can bring ideas to fruition to help yourself and possibly benefit others. During this time of unique importance in the world of medicine and science, Israel is a shining star in following the basic principle set forth in Deuteronomy: Choose Life. You can look at the what and the how of many ideas and inventions, but the vital why is at the core of medicine and biotechnology innovation—to improve and save lives.

With the results of interviews, emails, personal visits and extensive research, I will take you on a journey to explore how all this creative and outstanding innovation has happened. Come with me as we explore together the amazing, flourishing world of Israeli medicine and biotechnology.

Dr. Rob Norman

1

EMERGENCY MEDICINE

In the field of medical volunteer work, Israel leads the world in innovative services. United Hatzalah of Israel is the largest independent, non-profit, fully volunteer Emergency Medical Services organization that provides the fastest and free emergency medical first response throughout Israel. Using specially equipped motorcycle ambulances and a network of more than 2,500 volunteer medics, Hatzalah helps save thousands of lives each year across Israel. The group provides medical treatment in three minutes or less, a critical window of time between the onset of an emergency and the arrival of traditional ambulance assistance. As a designated national security asset by the Israel Defense Forces (IDF) Home Front Command, United Hatzalah's Life Compass Command Center's humanitarian services are free, universal and available 24 hours a day, seven days a week, 365 days a year, regardless of race, religion or national origin.

Eli Beer is the CEO of United Hatzalah. While working as a young Emergency Medical Technician (EMT) in Jerusalem, he recognized that heavy urban traffic and narrow streets often prevented ambulances from arriving in time to save a victim. He organized a volunteer unit of EMTs within his Jerusalem neighborhood. In 2006, after the Second Lebanon War, Beer brought together more than 50 separate Hatzalah chapters to form United Hatzalah of Israel. United Hatzalah pioneered the world's first ambucycles-- motorcycles equipped with a rear life-saving box that contains a complete trauma kit, an oxygen canister, a blood sugar monitor, and an automated external defibrillator. Each of the 440 ambucycles combines a driver and a vehicle agile enough to negotiate the busy traffic, obstructions, and narrow alleys of Israel.

United Hatzalah was started by a Hasidic Jew in

Williamsburg, Brooklyn. The group currently responds to approximately 800 calls per day. During large-scale emergencies such as the 2014 Israel–Gaza Conflict, the number jumps up to as many as 1,200 calls per day. In 2014, the organization answered more than 245,000 calls. Eli Beer presented a TedMed talk, in April 2013, titled, "The fastest ambulance? A motorcycle," in which he describes how he re-imagines first-response medicine by training volunteer EMTs to respond to local emergencies and stabilize victims until official help arrives. (https://www.ted.com/talks/eli_beer_the_fastest_ambul ance_a_motorcycle?).

The video has been viewed more than one million times to date. During his TedMed talk, Beer said "After we started our services in East Jerusalem, Jews were saving Arabs and Arabs were saving Jews. My own father had a heart attack and was saved by a Moslem Hatzalah driver." Of the volunteer medics, 38% are Haredi, 33.7% Modern Orthodox, 23.6% Secular, 3.1% Muslim, 1.1% Druze and .2% Christian, and .3% other.

Although United Hatzalah's lifesaving model has reduced average response time to three minutes, the average response time across Israel remains between 10 to 12 minutes. On sudden cardiac arrest calls—the best measure of emergency medical performance—United Hatzalah's success in reducing response times and increasing quality of care have changed in lockstep with national survival rates. According to the Israel Heart Society, in the 10 years since United Hatzalah's began, the rate of cardiac-arrest deaths has decreased by 50%. With 46.4 deaths per 100,000 people in terms of coronary-related mortality, the World Health Organization reports that Israel ranks 12th best out of 192 countries.

United Hatzalah partnered with Now Force to create a proprietary mobile dispatch application to receive calls, assess the unique capabilities, mobility and equipment of the closest volunteers, and then route the most appropriate medics to a given emergency. Today, the five closest volunteers receive alerts on their mobile phone through the Now Force command-and-control application and are guided on the fastest route.

During the high-profile abduction and murder of three Israeli youths in June 2014, United Hatzalah responded with SOS, a one-swipe emergency mobile alert application developed in conjunction with Now Force. SOS sends a distress signal to United Hatzalah's 24/7 dispatch center and transmits the user's GPS coordinates to law enforcement officials. The system replaces a process that may otherwise require days of legal maneuvering and functions as an emergency safety and security alert system, complementing direct verbal communication with police, fire, or medical emergency dispatchers.

Now Force raised $4.5 million in a Series B round of funding led by Verint Systems Inc. (NASDAQ: VRNT), along with the participation of current investors Winnovation, Indigo Strategic Holding LP and Monet Venture Group Limited. The company has expanded its offers with personal safety applications, cloud-based computer aided dispatch, and mobile response tools for campus security, private security, and public safety organizations. The app may be downloaded for free at sos.nowforce.com in both English and Hebrew.

Daniel Katzenstein, the Director of Marketing and Media for United Hatzalah, offered his comments on the technology and medicine scene in Israel. "If necessity is the mother of invention then self-reliance is the father and the culture of innovation is its incubator. Israel has been forced to rely on the intellectual capital of its human resources to compensate for its relative lack of natural resources as it struggles to survive in the region," Katzenstein said. "The outcome has been the technological advances that functions as force multipliers and resource optimizers in key survival fields such as military/security, water/agricultural and bio/med tech."

Pertaining to United Hatzalah, he added the company has "a very flat sense of hierarchy with that Israeli sense of openness that allows all elements of the organization to float their ideas towards management. If a field medic from Ashdod comes up with a better solution for a medical problem, the solution is rapidly evaluated internally tried and tested in the field and then either modified to final implementation or rejected. If a computer programmer comes up with an app or integration solution that can reduce response time and thereby save lives it will be fast-tracked in a real-world environment as quickly as possible."

I asked Katzenstein about Israeli military training as a springboard for science, technology, and medical innovation. "I would focus more on the mindset than the training. The Israeli military encourages innovative thinking in the problem-solving process from idea generation all the way through to implementation. With so much to risk if you are behind on the technology curve, calculated risk taking is encouraged. United Hatzalah's passion to find the fastest, highest quality and most efficient method to provide lifesaving emergency medical intervention is driven by a similar level of intensity. We have actively recruited and advanced key operational personnel from the ranks of relevant fields in the Israel Defense Forces (IDF)."

Israeli citizens utilize many of the new innovations created within its own healthcare environment such as United Hatzalah of Israel and provide financial and emotional support. "United Hatzalah is very close to the emergency healthcare end user particularly when they are in their most vulnerable stage, the moments after a terror attack, car accident or other medical emergency," Katzenstein said. "Once the citizens of Israel experienced near immediate emergency medical response due to the innovation of ambucycles, a revolutionary GPS colocation dispatch app and an intelligent distribution of committed volunteers responding from within the community, all stakeholders in the Israeli medical environment took notice and applauded its implementation. The grass-roots approach to overcome logistical, administrative and pessimistic obstacles was far more effective and faster than a formalized top-down approach."

What's in the future for United Hatzalah? "Right now, we are working on exporting our lifesaving model and technology to foreign countries. United Hatzalah of Panama was our first direct international adaptation in a Jewish community. Our activities and consultations in Brazil, Lithuania, India and others also bore significant impact. The current adaptation of United Hatzalah as United Rescue for the general community in Jersey City NJ has been an encouraging development and is a springboard to many other American and foreign cities interested in the model. If the light unto the nations we carry is a flashing red strobe so be it."

During the March 2015 American-Israel Public Affairs Committee (AIPAC) Policy Conference—the largest yearly gathering of the pro-Israel movement in the United States—United Hatzalah was honored as a featured innovator. AIPAC's Innovation Showcase was presented before 16,000 attendees and serves to highlight emerging technology developed in Israel but with worldwide impact. Eli Beer, on behalf of United Hatzalah, has received numerous international accolades, including the Israeli Presidential Award for Volunteerism in 2011 and the Institute of International Education's Victor J. Goldberg Prize in 2013.

"I guess you could call this a life-saving flash mob and it works. We all want to be heroes," Beer said. "We just need an innovative idea/ a promising idea, motivation and lots of chutzpah, and we can save millions of people that otherwise would not be saved."

I asked Beer what has set the scene for technology and medicine in Israel. "Israel, unfortunately, is disposed with endless challenges since its establishment until today," Beer said. "Unfortunately, in the past two decades, terrorism has challenged Israel and medical services in many ways, forcing us to think out of the box and find and create solutions to these challenges resulting in innovative technology, operational solutions and efficient implementation and execution."

During our discussion, I asked Beer about the distinctive characteristics of Israel in Medicine and Biotech that differentiates it from the rest of the world? Beer replied, "I think it goes back to the Start Up Nation, in High tech and Biotech. I think that the Israelis in general are thinking out of the box and after high school, they go to do their army service that puts the reality burden on them forcing them to think and operate more creatively, in an environment of creativity and innovation and not just standing by and waiting to see what happens. By nature, Israelis seek novel solutions/ fresh/ innovative solutions throughout all areas of life and Biotech is no exception. Beer offered his take on unique ways of coming up with creative solutions in his company. "Our organization is unique in that we provide emergency medical treatments on a community level," he said. "We always are looking for ways to minimize response times and maximize the treatment and care provided. We have both medical and IT people working together to develop both better medical solutions and technological logistical solutions."

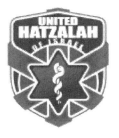

FRIENDS OF
UNITED HATZALAH
OF ISRAEL

"With the Israeli need to innovate since 1948, as the country was mostly desert, Israel has had a springboard to 'try', everything could be possible in a growing society and creativity has flourished," Beer said. "In the past 3 years over 80 companies were funded by one VC alone. There are many multiples of this figure with many buoyant buy outs."

I asked Beer about the necessity of underground operating rooms at Hadassah hospital and other medical centers. Beer replied, "Reality, very simple. Every 2-3 years, there is a war in which mortars and missiles are shot all over Israeli, from up north in Lebanon or in the south from Gaza, making the Israeli home front a place regularly under attack. Underground shelters and operating rooms have been built to protect the people in

Israel and continue with operations as normal during such attacks."

When asked about the most important things he is working on right now, Beer replied, "Saving lives," he said. "And bringing response rates from three minutes to 90 seconds."

2

DISABILITY AND REHABILITATION

Walking into the ReWalk headquarter Yokneam Ilit, Israel, I had little understanding of what I was to experience and how much it would change my world. When I was in medical school, I had spent six weeks in training at the Rehabilitation Institute of Chicago and remembered the intense struggles and depression of those that had lost the use of their lower extremities due to severe spinal cord injury. No longer able to walk, the only option was the use of wheelchairs for mobility.

We were touring on the first Doctors for Israel mission, part of the Jewish National Fund, primarily physicians in different specialties from all over the United States. As I looked around, I noted the amazed expressions on the faces of my colleagues.

A middle–aged man in a wheelchair volunteered to demonstrate for our group. He was a dark-haired man with stocky features, and rose from his wheelchair to balance on the ReWalk exoskeleton. Each of us looked on with great anticipation. He gracefully lifted himself and strapped himself in. Within a few moments he was walking. I thought I was on a science fiction movie set.

Think about it. Put yourself in the situation of someone with a profound disability that results in lower extremity paralysis. You will probably experience depression and a vastly lower quality of life than in your previous life. Of course, you will probably have a strong desire to walk again and be eye to eye with peers in social interactions. Your wheelchair allows only limited community access and inhibits meaningful social roles in the community. And then you find out about a modern technology/ recent technology called robotic exoskeletons that would allow you and others with spinal cord injury to walk.

In 2014, ReWalk Robotics Ltd. (NASDAQ: RWLK) had a major German insurance company be the first to reimburse a ReWalk system for personal use and insurers across the globe have followed with reimbursement policies for ReWalk's exoskeleton technology. The German ReWalker who had his ReWalk Personal system reimbursed by this insurance company had been confined to a wheelchair because of a car accident in 1999. The accident caused a complete Spinal Cord Injury (SCI) at the Thoracic 8 level and rendered him paraplegic. He saw the ReWalk exoskeleton demonstrated at a trade show and contacted the company to inquire and eventually successfully completed the required eligibility review that allowed approval for the reimbursement of a ReWalk Personal system.

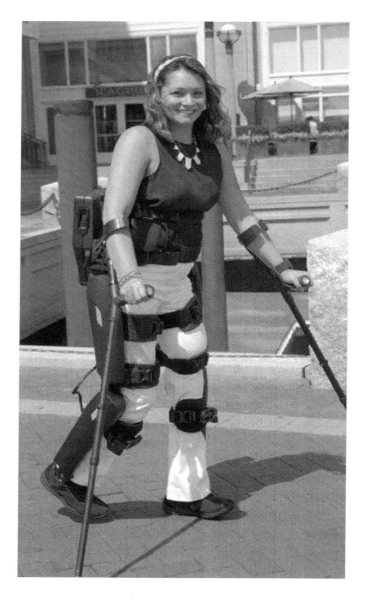

http://rewalk.com/rewalk-personal-3

The ReWalk Rehabilitation model currently is used by patients in rehab centers all over the world. ReWalk is a wearable robotic exoskeleton that provides powered hip and knee motion to enable individuals with spinal cord injury. Sensors in the device detect subtle shifts in the user's center of gravity and upper-body movements and automatically translate these shifts into movement of its motorized leg joints. The ReWalk device allows the user to stand upright, walk, turn, and climb and descend stairs. The new model—the Personal 6.0--is worn outside the clothing and is attached to the user via leg braces and a harness and provides a more precise custom-fit system. In addition to the ability to stand and walk independently, clinical studies of the ReWalk Rehabilitation system show significant potential physiological benefits. It is the only FDA cleared exoskeleton for rehabilitation and personal use in the United States and is the most used and studied exoskeleton technology of its kind, with hundreds of ReWalkers worldwide.

The visit to Rewalk changed my life, and I wanted to learn more about how Israel made this happen? Was this just an exceptional outcome? Hardly, I soon found out, and over the next two years I have discovered an amazing world in Israel.

ApiFix, a Treadlines company, was awarded Best Start-Up 2012 by Israel's Office of the Chief Scientist of the Ministry of Economy for a less invasive, less painful, and less costly option for spine curvature correction. Apifix is developing a truly breakthrough minimally invasive deformity correction system for patients with Adolescent Idiopathic Scoliosis (AIS).

Today's gold standard for correcting spinal deformities involves fusing an average of 10 motion levels using many screws in a surgical procedure that lasts an average of six hours and costs upward of $100,000. As opposed to the current procedure, ApiFix uses only two screws to support its ratchet-based, small expandable rod inserted through a small incision in the patient's back. In addition to the smaller incision, a shortened surgery time (1 hour vs. 4-6 hours) and reduced hospitalization stay.

I interviewed Uri Arnin, Founder and CEO and chief innovator of ApiFix Ltd. about the success of his company and the distinctive characteristics of the Israeli biotech cluster. "We have close communication between companies of the same field and willingness to assist each other. The same subcontractors and advisers support similar companies and help to share the experience," Arnin said. "We have a fast turnaround of production cycles, due to personal relationship with suppliers."

When asked about the speed of innovation, Arnin said, "The first R&D cycles are being performed in Israel, 'quick and dirty'. The pivotal tests and validations are being done abroad. In today's world, it is quite easy to use infrastructure abroad and get its reputation."

I asked him about obstacles to success for his and other companies. "It is very different from one company to the other," Arnin said. "In my case the FDA is the biggest obstacle. Not because of the demands but because the long timeline, inflated cost/excessive cost/prohibitive cost and uncertainty. Investors are now afraid to invest in breakthrough technologies just because of that. As a summary, I am not optimistic at all about that space. The regulatory atmosphere (mainly FDA) becomes more and more difficult. The prices are going down and the investors have more attractive options to double their money. As a main single comment, the FDA is simply killing the innovation in the field of medical devices."

I wondered if the robust growth/sturdy growth in Israel's high-tech sector only benefits a small part of the Israeli population. Armin replied, "Most of the money invested in my companies came from the US and most of it was spent in Israel. That means jobs and work for many people."

I asked him about the quality of Israeli subcontractors and outsourcing. "In my case," Armin said, "Most of the subcontractors used are on a top level when compared to US and EU, where I had the chance to visit many times. Only when dealing with very unique issues, like micro motors or special ceramic coating, I had to use overseas sourcing."

Over the years I had read about the importance of the military as a training ground for science, technology, and medicine. Armin's response took me in a new direction. "In my experience, the army teaches you that nothing is impossible. It teaches you that timing is critical. It teaches you that even when everything goes against you, going forwards is the way to win. It is the commando spirit that is important, not the physical things."

As noted, an open and honest evaluation of innovation along with the "Commando spirit" provides a positive attitude and work incentive to not give up and succeed Armin stated, "In the field of medical devices most of the ventures fail, for one reason or another. People simply go on to the next one, hoping it will work this time, with more experience and better understanding. If you fail two times your third venture may be much better. In Israel, it is not a shame to fail."

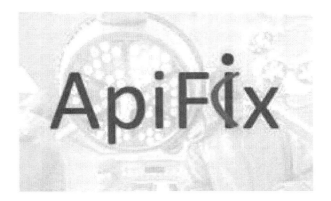

Minimally invasive device for treating AIS or adolescent idiopathic scoliosis

What is it about the Israeli culture that drives the country to grow in biotechnology? What makes this culture different from other? The Israelis may have learned or imitated previous people but so do other cultures. Why does this happen in such a unique way here? Does the need for innovation fuel a cross-fertilization that is greater than the sum of its parts?

"It is the ability to share experience and information that makes a difference. When I have a problem, I can call a mate from another company in my field and get most of the help he can give," Armin said. "I am helping people from other companies all the time. No money change hands. The same is true to every employee in the company, each coming with a unique experience/distinct experience. So, when you have a company with 10 employees they cover a 'net of information' there a superiority or inferiority complex? Is the fact they are surrounded by enemies and already an underdog work in a David and Goliath manner? "Yes, in a way," Armin stated. "I have no fear to approach Medtronic or J&J and tell them 'I am doing better than you in this area.' I know that being big means also being fat and slow."

What about language barriers? Armin replied, "The only problem is in the US, where speaking in the "wrong" accent is many times close to a crime…"

How has Israel instituted technology to help with understanding dealing with various societies and cultures? Are these practices currently being taught in the schools and colleges?

"Not really," Armin said. "If you are interested you can learn from other colleagues. Basically, once you respect the other side and once you come with solid science, there is no problem."

I asked Armin to describe the healthcare environment in Israel and the utilization of any of the new innovations. "My market is the US and the EU. Israel has no real meaning when practicing the new technology. The only upside here is the ability to get real and direct feedback on what you do."

The key issue, of course, is funding, which comes from various sources, including the Israeli government and the United States government. "The first funding from the government is critical for success. It is small

($0.5M) but easy to get," Armin said. "The next funding comes usually from the US. You have to do it yourself and this is the most difficult part in the company life. Today it is so much easier to start a new venture in the US. You can get more money with better terms. Also, your ability to raise the next round is better as a lot of investors would never invest over the ocean."

Now is a very unique time in the history of innovation in Israel. Armin said, "In my mind, the main thing that made the change, around 20 years ago, was the internet. The ability to have access to the same information (Science, Patents, Commercial, etc.) just like an American scientist has made it possible for people in Israel to participate in the game. Then, our ability to do it faster and cheaper made us attractive for some investors."

Much has been written and said about the Israeli personality, and I asked Armin about it. "Israelis are so much different from each other. There is nothing common you can tell about them. In a very general way you can say that they are very open and clear. You will hear from them exactly what they think, right on the spot, if you ask them or not... People may like or dislike that.

When talking with Americans, many times I go out of a long meeting having no idea what they really think," Armin said.

I asked Armin about the most important thing he's working on right now. "I am working on a revolutionary way to correct scoliosis, using everything I have learned along my life and especially the experience in the spine field I have gained along the last 12 years. The hardest decision I've made so far is to start this venture and not do something else." I asked Armin about the greatest obstacles he has had thus far and what he perceives to be some of the obstacles he will encounter in the future. "The answer for both is the same," Armin replied. "It is the very conservative way spine surgeons think and behave. The terms Innovative, Revolutionary and First of its kind may sound good but in the real spine field it is very difficult to introduce new things. They will always ask for a five year follow up and would always prefer someone else help with that."

Who takes care of the disabled in Israel?

Of course, there are many wonderful providers for the

disabled in Israel. One location that stands out is the Aleh Negev-Nahalat Eran, a state-of-the-art rehabilitative village in the northern Negev near Ofakim that offers unparalleled care for people with severe disabilities. Major General (Res.) Doron Almog is the chairman of ALEH Negev. He is an Israeli military hero whose severely disabled son, Eran, was ALEH Negev's first resident. Eran was the spirit and inspiration for the founding of the Village, and following his untimely passing in February 2007, the village was renamed ALEH Negev-Nahalat Eran as a tribute and legacy.

Aleh Negev is a village in every sense of the word and is currently home to over 140 young people who are encouraged to develop a greater degree of independence in order to become productive members of Israeli society. At full capacity the village has the ability to care for 230 residents and has 12,000 outpatient treatments annually. As the center's web site states, the village "provides residential care for children with severe disabilities as they grow from adolescents into young adults, and empowers them to interact with the outside world, develop a greater degree of independence and live quality lives while realizing their full potential." Before Aleh Negev was built, patients had to wait several months for therapy sessions in the existing local medical center or travel up to four hours to medical centers to the Tel Aviv area. In addition, Aleh Negev provides jobs to hundreds of area residents in education, rehabilitation, maintenance, administration, medicine, supportive care and more. Aleh Negev-Nahalat Eran has connected Israeli government ministries, foundations, philanthropists and individuals worldwide in a project creating hope and flourishing opportunities for integration, understanding and acceptance of people with disabilities within society at large.

Aleh Negev, a $42 million-dollar National Project for the State of Israel, is the only facility of its kind in Israel and is being closely studied by experts from around the world as the paradigm of excellence in rehabilitative care. A major new Rehabilitation and Neurological Hospital is also being built.

I must mention one more program that is incredibly important and innovative. "Special in Uniform" is an innovative program that integrates youth with disabilities into the Israel Defense Forces (IDF) and helps prepare them for careers following army service. The program was founded "to give everyone a right to fulfill their potential and be accepted into society, regardless of any disability" and helps its graduates integrate into the workforce and Israeli society. The special needs soldiers would have been rejected until a few years ago, and now there are 350 soldiers with special needs serving in 22 army bases across Israel in a unit named "Special in Uniform."

At the most recent JNF annual conference in Hollywood, Florida, we heard a powerful talk by Maj. Riki Golan. She is a young officer whose father was decorated for bravery in the Yom Kippur War, and she was born with a breathing defect that affected her ability to walk. In fact, the doctors told her parents that she would never walk. Her father refused to give in and would not allow her to give in. He taught her to be stubborn, and although it is not easy, she walks – and she can walk unaided. She said that she is grateful to be allowed to serve her country.

Let me shift to another military narrative that is quite

amazing and reflective of Israel's commitment to peace.
During my most recent trip to Israel in March of 2017,
our group from JNF's Doctors for Israel visited Ziv
Hospital, at the bottom of Safed. The hospital is a
government public general hospital with 310 beds that
treats patients from the Upper Galilee and the northern
Golan. Ziv serves as a Regional Trauma Center in case of
accidents, natural disaster, terror attacks and war. The
hospital serves the local Jewish kibbutzim, moshavim and
small towns as well as the local Arab and Druze villages.
Walking the halls, you may hear Hebrew, Arabic, Russian,
Amharic or English being spoken and translated.

We were able to meet with three wounded Syrian
soldiers that were being treated for free in the hospital.
After six years of civil war, healthcare in Syria is almost
destroyed. It has been reported that there are only seven
doctors and about a million people live in the border
areas. Syria has been at war with Israel since May 1948
and these wounded men were our enemies.

With the help of an Arabic-speaking social worker,
Fares, we learned the story of each of them. For security
reasons, each soldier was unable to contact any family

member to provide a current location. Despite an isolation from their previous life, each expressed tremendous appreciation for the life-saving help they were receiving. The youngest of the three had suffered a leg amputation and was awaiting a donated prosthesis prior to getting out and being dropped off at the border. He told me he had 12 siblings, all soldiers, and that he was going to go back to fight against the Assad regime when he was released.

The treated Syrian patients do not do follow-up at Ziv and the expensive devices such as prothesis are not returned. The hospital absorbs the cost, an unavoidable expense of treating Syrian patients. The care is paid for by the Israeli government, Ziv Medical Center itself, and by individual contributions to Ziv. Contributions to Ziv are tax-deductible in both the US and Israel. (Friends of Ziv Medical Center, Inc. is a registered 501(c)(3) charity.)

The IDF will take back them back to the border and send them home once they recover, as they have with more than 800 patients they have treated. Upon leaving, each patient is given a summary of their medical treatment, written in Arabic on plain paper that does not indicate treatment in Israel.

Dr. Lerner and Dr. Salman Zarka are attending physicians at Ziv and wrote the book Complicated War Trauma and Care of the Wounded: The Israeli Experience in Medical Care and Humanitarian Support of Syrian refugees (Springer). The book includes orthopedics and other surgical treatment, psychological therapy, and ethical issues involved in treating enemy soldiers and civilians.

I will be forever touched by the people I met at Ziv Hospital; their work is a shining example of Tikkun Olam.

3

DECREASING DRUG COSTS

Daniel A. Goldstein, MD, is a Senior Physician in Medical Oncology at the Rabin Medical Center in Israel. I spoke to Dr. Goldstein about building economic models that are cost-effective, particularly with oncology drugs. He and his colleagues built economic models and published in high-end medical journals such as the Journal of Clinical Oncology (see references) The studies were reported in the Wall Street Journal, Washington Post, and in the New York Times.

"I grew up in England and went to medical school in England," Goldstein said. "I met my wife in Israel. She's from New York. I ended up in New York where I did my residency. Later I did a fellowship in hematology and medical oncology at Emory. During that time, I was also involved in doing research in health economics and understanding the cost effectiveness and value of cancer drugs. Then from there, it had always been a dream of mine to move to Israel with my family, my wife and two children at the time. We recently had a third baby."

"Why Israel?"

"I have family here. I'd always felt it was the ultimate home for me. I've been in many places. I grew up in England. I lived in America for 9 years. I also worked and traveled in India, Africa, Europe, and ultimately, I felt my home was in Israel. I was doing work on the health system or economics related to the US healthcare system. It was ultimately quite an attractive idea to do work based on the Israeli healthcare system."

"And what about your transition to Israel?"

"In Israel, I started working at the Rabin Medical Center, treating patients with cancer and additionally developing further economic analyses based on the Israeli system, and still working on the US system as well as other countries in the world. The aim of it was try to understand some of those many, many new drugs that are being brought to the market and trying to understand which drugs should be paid for and which drugs shouldn't be paid for based on what phase of data is available from the clinical trials."

The Davidoff Center at the Rabin Medical Center in Petah Tikvah is one of the most sophisticated and innovative facilities in the Middle East for the treatment of malignant diseases and is estimated to provide comprehensive medical treatment to over 16% of Israel's cancer patients. The unique Center consolidates under one roof all of Rabin Medical Center's oncology and hemato-oncology inpatient facilities and outpatient services.

"What other items do you look at?'" I asked.

"We try to understand what appropriate prices should be for these drugs when they hit the marketplace. What the appropriate approval process should be, or develop a method of value-based prices, where we would figure out based on the efficacy the drug demonstrates, actually developing a price based on the efficacy."

"What about now?"

"I'm now working with heads of hospitals in Israel as well as advising heads of Health Maintenance Organization (HMOs) as well, about many issues related to cancer drugs. I have a unique position in the fact that I've worked in several different systems in the world. Coming from the UK, I was brought up with a single-payer system which has many problems, but also has many advantages. Then I was challenged by moving to the US where I saw a different system where there were, again, many benefits or many things that were better than the UK but also many things that were worse than in the UK."

"What did you learn along the way when you studied the American health system? How did it compare to the Israeli system?" I asked.

"Those experiences challenged me to realize that there actually is no perfect system. It helped me to understand some of the benefits and problems. Sometimes you can get better care in America but obviously one of the biggest issues before the Affordable Care Act came in, we found that were huge portions of the population who didn't get healthcare. Whereas in England perhaps one may argue that sometimes the quality of care isn't quite as good but the fact that they're giving care to everybody is definitely a huge advantage. Then having had that background and coming to Israel, I see a new system. There's pros and cons of every system. Hopefully, having been in a few different systems I have the maturity to realize that most systems have both advantages and disadvantages."

"It sounds quite useful to have somebody who is a clinician to be able to do what you do," I said. "What's the way that you analyze the data and how is it unique in your process?"

"What we do is build economic models which are cost-effectiveness analyses that are essentially a marriage of publicly available data from clinical trials merging together with cost data," Goldstein said. "In the US, they're building it into a computerized mathematical model to then understand the value or the cost effectiveness of each individual drug. This was, to a certain extent, unique in America because people have been doing these cost-effectiveness studies for a while in many different countries. They're used in Canada and England and several other countries to guide coverage of if a drug should be approved or not. However, the problem in the United States was the fact that there is no evaluation of value. The FDA approves drugs based purely based on safety and efficacy and has no mandate to evaluate cost or value."

"What happens once they are approved?

"Medicare has to provide any drugs that are approved. They're not allowed to negotiate their price. Essentially what's happened is the drug prices have been rising and rising over the past several years. You now have a situation where pretty much most of the new cancer drugs that enter the marketplace cost around about $15,000 per month. The price is no way linked to the efficacy or to the benefit of the drug. Sometimes you have a drug that may cure patients and it's $15,000 a month, or you may have a drug that just increases life for 6 weeks, but the patients still die. Essentially, we developed these economic models to understand the value and the cost and efficacy of different drugs. We've used it as a tool to suggest that some of these drugs should be a lot cheaper than what they actually are."

"Have you developed new models to prove your point?" I asked.

"In the model that we did most recently, that there was much interest in, we took a drug that we were expected to get approved but wasn't yet approved by the FDA, a drug for Stage IV lung cancer. We did effectively a backwards model where we estimated how much the drug should cost if it gets approved for it be considered cost effective. We did this analysis and that got published in JAMA Oncology. That was reported in the Wall Street Journal and a bunch of various places to try to put a certain amount of pressure to the pharmaceutical industry to price it at an appropriate price related to the benefit the drug provides."

"When was it that you started to look at all this cost data? When did you start getting so interested in efficacy and cost?" I asked.

"It was a kind of gradual process. I've always been very interested in cost. I was always interested in the bigger picture. I was never really a basic scientist. Then when I was at Emory, I was given the opportunity to study it more deeply and then I started to do these studies myself. I think we published maybe 10 papers in the couple years."

"What is it different in Israel?" I asked. "How are they unique? Are they more open in Israel to cutting costs? Any reasons that they can cut costs that you couldn't do in the United States?"

"I think the main difference is between countries is based essentially in culture. I think in America there's the notion that everything should be available and there's no price that's too high. This kind of cultural feeling has enabled the prices to become inflated. Whereas in countries like Israel which is more practical where they say, no we have a budget. This is the budget. This is all there is. New drugs that come along, they get evaluated for the benefit they provide. There's an estimation of how much it will cost to treat all the patients with that disease with that particular drug than the consideration of what the benefit actually is. Then a calculation to say whether or the not the country can afford it or not."

"When does this occur?"

"Every year there is an analysis on new drugs that try to enter what is called 'The Basket.' There's maybe 100 new drugs that are trying to get into the basket that the companies are pushing to get approved. They get analyzed and each one gets marked a number of points based on what level of efficacy it gives and what the disease is, and then there's a calculation to say what it's actually going to cost and if we actually have the money to pay for it."

"Quite practical," I said.

"They're practical here. In England they're practical, but they also make an estimation of value. They say, look, there's a point at which something is too expensive and it's not giving us enough benefit. Whereas in America, there's been a cultural notion that there is no point that's too high. Essentially industry has taken advantage of this and they've just inflated the prices. Drugs in America cost significantly more than drugs cost in the rest of the world."

"We hear stories here all the time like you mentioned of drugs now going sky high. In my field, in dermatology, when they decide about a biologic, let's say there are five biologics to treat psoriasis, and a new one comes out. Well, it's kind of uncanny unless you have your insight into it. If it's something like a Biologic New that's only given prescribed 4 times a year versus an Enbrel which maybe 2 x week. Well, it's kind of uncanny to an outsider to think, they more than coincidental came up with this price of $20,000 a year to match the amount for Biologic A. Now we don't know behind the scenes if it really costs them that much or they're just making a bigger margin because of it. For you, that's probably an obvious fact. We see this all the time.

"What about vaccines? I have done a lot of work in public health. Public health focuses heavily on safe food and drinking water, sanitation, antibiotics and vaccines. I think that continues the vaccine route. What do you think is going to happen next?" I asked.

"First of all, I love the fact about what you said about

public health. I also have a public health background. You're totally right. Clean water. Many of these drugs that we use now, they really make very minimal incremental benefit. The biggest health changes of the 20th and 19th century was just simply having clean sanitation and clean water. Vaccines fall under the realm of immunotherapy and is a very exciting field right now within cancer. There are several/many new drugs that are coming out particularly in melanoma treatments and some already approved. Many vaccines have been tried in cancer but haven't had remarkable success so far. If there's going to be anything more in the future, I don't know. I'm not I don't see a lot of cancer vaccines in the pipeline, but many new immunotherapy agents. The PD-1 inhibitors, or PDL-1 inhibitors, such as Nivolumab (Opdivo) and Pembrolizumab (Keytruda), those are the really exciting drugs that we are talking about now that have been approved."

4

PREVENTING ERRORS

I interviewed Gidi Stein, MD, Ph.D. the co-founder of MedAware and a professor of medicine and molecular imaging at Tel Aviv University in Israel. According to the MedAware website, "Healthcare providers, payers and pharmacy chains can leverage on their big data to identify and eliminate a wide range of prescription errors and provide better risk management." The web promotional information, in summary, states "MedAware's process saves many lives, reduces unnecessary hospital costs, improves patient safety and satisfaction and improves overall healthcare efficiency and quality."

Stein noted that several years prior to beginning the company, "I came across a tragic case of a nine-year-old Israeli boy who died because his primary-care physician accidentally prescribed the wrong drug. The ease with which a little boy died because of a mistaken click of a button was horrifying to me as a physician and as a parent. We founded MedAware in order to try and prevent such cases."

With the rapid increase in Electronic Health Records (EHRs) and computerized prescription orders, medication errors are gaining more attention. The journal BMJ Quality and Safety included a study of more than 1 million medication errors reported to the U.S. Pharmacopeia MEDMARX reporting system between 2003 and 2010. More than 63,000 of the errors were related to computerized provider-order entry. More than 3.7 billion retail prescriptions are filled annually in the US, and 1.5 million preventable errors result in death or injury along with billions in wasteful health care spending.

How does this drive for innovation work? What has set the scene for technology and medicine in Israel? Stein replied, "A few years ago, Shimon Peres, Israel's president, visited the House of Lords in London and was asked, "What is the secret of Jewish/Israeli entrepreneurship?" His answer was: "Chronic discontent". When asked about distinctive characteristics of the Israeli biotech cluster that drives it, Stein included, "Low funds and hunger for making a meaningful impact and making a difference."

One Israeli development has been the creation of underground operating rooms at Hadassah Hospital and other medical centers. I had a tour of the Hadassah facilities during a recent trip to Israel and saw first-hand the 20 ultra-modern operating rooms in the Sarah Wetsman Davidson Hospital four floors underground, with built-in safeguards to handle biological or chemical attacks. Stein said, "The reality is that once every few years Israel is engaged in battle, and recently these wars include vast missile attacks throughout the country. This necessitates building secure environments to provide continuous care to civilians."

I asked Stein if there is typically one innovator or a group of people working together in innovation in his company. "We are a small early-stage startup, we are all innovators... we are a multi-disciplinary team trying to solve real-world problems with practical and cutting-edge technology. The word 'impossible' does not live in our offices," Stein said. "The drivers to Israeli innovation include: If someone says it's impossible – we must prove him wrong, hunger, and not being afraid to fail. We often don't teach or learn how to innovate, we just do it...fail... and do it again..."

Israel excels in innovation readiness but appears to be lacking in physical infrastructure. What is it about the Israeli culture, despite its limitations, that drives the country to grow in biotechnology? Stein responded, "This drives innovation to areas where physical infrastructure is not critical, such as software, algorithms, security, cyber and others. Bio-technology is an area where you need relatively limited resources but strong brains to innovate, and a multidisciplinary approach, which is our strongpoint, usually wins."

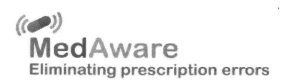

I asked Stein if there has there been an immigration policy to recruit more scientists, physicians, and researchers. "Following the Holocaust, Israel was founded and left its doors open for all Jewish immigrants from around the world. This brought to Israel bright scientists from the US and Europe, and in the last 30 years, from the former Soviet Union," Stein said.

One of the major challenges Israel is facing right now is the improvement of its productivity rates to strengthen its overall competitiveness. "In Israel, there are large (and growing) populations who do not contribute to the work force and shift the GDP downwards," Stein said. "Although this does not affect my company in the short term, it would definitely have a grim effect on the prospects of growth if left unattended by the government."

Military training is known as a strong springboard for science, technology, and medical innovation. "The Israeli military has a long tradition of innovation. Most of the soldiers are young and bright and try to make a difference for the safety of their families. This environment nourishes many ideas and innovations, which causes 19-

year-olds to be responsible for multi-million-dollar operational projects, while trying all the time to make them better. In many cases, they are not aware that something is impossible to achieve, so they just do it," Stein said.

Stein added, "Although conservative, Israel's healthcare environment is very open to innovation, mainly because it is quite centralized and NOT private, thus we try to focus on the best healthcare we can provide our patients and not necessarily the profit/cost."

I asked Stein about language barriers when dealing with so many various countries.

"We talk with our hands... it's easier to understand," he said.

Why is this time so unique in the history of medicine in Israel and for MedAware?

"This is the time we can finally harness big data of electronic medical records, for which Israel has unique decades of documented electronic history, to provide personalized medicine and advance research. We are saving lives by identifying and eliminating prescription errors using big data analytics. Israeli innovation and technology had brought cheap and safe circumcision, as HIV preventive measure, to Africa (http://prepex.com/)."

For funding, Stein and others often mention the Chief Scientist Office grants, angel investors, venture capital, and joining with companies in the US and elsewhere. I asked him about financial incentives. "In recent years, there have been changes in the Chief Scientist Office and there are many incentives for high-tech and life-science companies, which facilitates growth." As far as obstacles to growth, he included "funding, engaging customers, and creating strategic relationships outside Israel."

I asked Stein if he could describe the pros and cons of dealing with Israelis and their personalities. "Pros: we usually say what we think. Cons: we usually say what we think."

5

ACCELERATORS AND INCUBATORS

Todd Dollinger is Chairman and CEO of The Trendlines Group.

"How did you get involved with your company? What were you doing before and what made you gravitate towards this?" I asked.

"The beginning of Trendlines actually dates back all the way to the US. I've been in Israel since 1990, so I've been over here for 27 years now. In the States, I worked in business development and sales, and that company was known as Trendlines. My first job in Israel in 1991 was working for a startup medical device company. We were developing processed EEG for monitoring depth of anesthesia. That was my introduction to the medical device industry. The truth is, until I moved to Israel, I didn't know there was a medical device industry."

"You didn't know until you moved to Israel?"

"I didn't know there was one anywhere. I was completely ignorant. So, for me, it was a wholly new industry, a wholly new opportunity. And so, in 1993, my now business partner, Steve Rhodes and I left that company, and we started Trendlines here in Israel. It began as a business development firm, and a very important part of our business was working with startup medical device companies. That morphed over the years, and in 2007, with extensive experience working with startups, we started The Trendlines Group as an investment company. We acquired two Israeli government-franchised business incubators, and that's what we've been doing – and growing – ever since. We have been very involved in startups since the 1990's, and have been involved in the medical device industry in Israel and worldwide since that time."

"How does one go about acquiring government incubators as you mentioned?" I asked.

"I'll give you the short version of a long story. But to try and make it a reasonable length, I'll go back to when I made Aliyah – when I moved to Israel – and you'll remember very well that at that time there was tremendous Russian immigration occurring. The Former Soviet Union (FSU) had come apart and Jews who had not previously been allowed to leave the FSU emigrated, with many coming to Israel. I made Aliyah in 1990 from the State of Kansas, so my wife and I and our three little girls were the "Great Kansas Aliyah Wave" of 1990. But that was around the same time as the massive FSU immigration, and one of the things that the government did was to establish business incubators to create jobs. And that jobs creation work was really focused on the new immigrants from the FSU. It was just a fascinating time, with these really, really driven people, people who had come here to escape the Soviet Union, and were trying to figure out how to move from one mindset, from one economy, from one culture, to something so completely different."

"An exciting time," I said.

"Right. So, the government set up this system of business incubators, which interestingly, was quite different from the American model in one very, very important way. And that was, if you came into an Israeli Government-licensed business incubator, it meant that there was an investment being made into your startup. Now, it was a small investment, but it made all the difference. And the American model, and the model worldwide, except for Israel at that time was, in business incubation, there wasn't an investment that was attached to your joining an incubator. You were going to some building that the local government had remodeled, and there was some former city government official who was now running it. It was just a chance to rent offices and be with some other startups. But in Israel, the model was different, and we became involved with that from very early on. In the very beginning, all the incubators were non-profit, which was very appropriate because, in the first years, none of them made a profit."

"All run by government people?" I asked.

"The incubators were owned by universities and other non-profits. But things started to happen and some of the companies that got started began to succeed, learning from the failures that preceded them. Some raised money, some brought products to market, some went public, some were sold to large corporations or went public. With this, Israel's incubator system began to really firm up and to strengthen. And then, there were other changes. The government again came in and made changes, including privatizing the incubator system. In the privatization process, we acquired two of those incubators. Today, it's very difficult to win the government licenses. We had to compete for renewal of our license for Trendlines Incubators Israel; companies seeking licenses in that same tender included Medtronic, GE, IBM, Boston Scientific, and more. They were competing for one of the same licenses that we won for an additional eight years. Medtronic, by the way, also won a license in partnership with IBM; it's tremendously competitive to get these licenses now."

"So, you own one of them?"

"Yes. Under our Trendlines Incubators Israel license,

we invest in the life sciences, operating as Trendlines Medical and Trendlines Agtech, which of course, invests in agricultural technology. Our investments are in the life sciences and only in these two areas; we're very mission-focused. Quite simply, we create and develop companies to improve the human condition. And with that as our mission, it drives us to focus on medical and agricultural technologies."

"And then you had these very competitive situations after it was privatized to get these licenses? And it's grown more competitive over time?"

"Absolutely... Much more so," Dollinger said, "and we are Israel's leading life sciences investor, having started and invested in 10 new companies in Israeli in 2016."

"They still do the startups. They might not get the licensing right away but they're growing as many startups." Perhaps to delete? I don't understand.

"You bet. Part of that is through Israel's incubator system. Part of that is by the fact that in addition to, or directly related to the fact there's so many startups, is we also have one of the most sophisticated venture capital industries in the world, second only to the US, which is just stunning, of course. As you know, our population is only 8.5 million, and yet we're second largest in venture capital and third largest in terms of number of companies traded on NASDAQ."

"If you look back to 1990, to where you are now, could you have imagined this, or did you see it from an earlier stage heading in this direction?" I asked.

"When I came here I saw none of this coming. None of it. I came to Israel because this is where I wanted to live, and this is where my wife and I decided that we wanted to raise our children. I sold my business in the US, we sold the house, we sold the cars and we came over here with no idea as to what the future would bring. Candidly, the advent of the internet, the former Soviet Union coming apart allowing the Russian Aliyah – these things coming together, all at the same time causes Israel to truly blossom as a place business for the world to do business. Partly because of changes made by the government, partly because it was the right time, remarkable things happened. The Israeli economy was a disaster in the mid '80s with hyper-inflations and host of structural problems but, by the end of the '80s, Israel was really beginning to develop the economic stability necessary to become the developed country that Israel is today."

"But you were out there witnessing an amazing time. Literally one of the most amazing times in world economy, I think," I said.

"Oh, you bet."

"That's why I'm so passionate about the opportunities that Israel represents."

"Well, of course, you should be. High level of importance. Start-up Nation, it's famous, and it's really helped brand Israel. As I said to one of the authors not that long ago, "Your book was the greatest single piece of propaganda for the State of Israel since Leon Uris wrote Exodus. I'm not sure he liked the word 'propaganda', but I think he appreciated the compliment."

"What about the overall quality of health care?"

"Israel certainly ranks among the top. There are very real differences between how medical services are delivered here versus the general privatized system in the US. If you look at the major HMOs in the US you'll find a fair number of similarities. But I believe that the quality of care is generally quite similar. And here we have what's principally a government-sponsored HMO system, where the HMOs compete. And then a small amount of private medicine on top of it."

"Jon Medved is a prime mover in channeling the innovative energy in Israel. Where along the line did you guys meet?" I asked.

"I've known Jon for more than 20 years. And Jon, of course, has created what is clearly the most important crowdfunding organization in the world, equity crowdfunding, more specifically. OurCrowd is an investor in Trendlines. They invested in Trendlines and one of our companies as well. OurCrowd helps draw attention to Trendlines, as does our annual company showcase and our AgriVest conference; both our conferences draw delegations from around the world with attendees listening to our companies present and talk about investing and doing business."

"So why your success?"

"Innovation management and entrepreneurial spirit – that's why Trendlines is so successful. I'm not an inventor, and I'm not a technology guy. But Trendlines has become expert at managing innovation, managing early-stage investing risk, and in establishing business models that work for multiple parties, not just for an investor, not just for an entrepreneur, but for everyone."

"What drives innovation in Israel?"

"Israel has become known for, and not just known for, but truly successful as innovators. Part of it relates to our being Jews, and the history this brings. Our history is most assuredly not a story of only happy days, but, rather, a history that forces us into the position of needing to be innovators, needing to be independent. This drive for independence causes a need for innovation. Jewish tradition and Jewish education are true drivers; while the modern State of Israel only dates to 1948, the history of the Jews encompasses thousands of years. I was in China a couple of weeks ago, and had this conversation with some of my Chinese friends. Most religions teach from the point of view of dogma, such as, "This is the knowledge, memorize it, know it, understand it, bring it into your heart." The Jewish approach is people sitting and discussing the Torah, discussing what the rabbis have said about it, and arguing about it; we're talking about students being taught, being invited to argue with this rabbi. Now, you're not going to see that in China. You're not going see an engineer working in a company, arguing with the CEO. Not true in Israel. That's welcomed at Trendlines. Everybody's arguing with everybody. Someone's yelling at someone else, and that's OK. When it comes to figuring out latest ways to do things, I think that this concept that you must be open to new ideas, you must learn how to argue, you must know how to present your concept, and you need to listen to the others, if for no other reason so that you can argue with them; this is tremendously important to innovation. Dogma does not help innovation; challenging ideas are necessary for innovation."

"The comparison to China is particularly useful," I said. "Both cultures are very ambitious and education-oriented."

"You're 100% right. Let me put a fine point on it. Interestingly, Jews have some similarities with the Chinese. We are a couple of ancient cultures, the Chinese and the Jews, and a couple of new states, Israel from 1948 and the Republic of China only from 1949. Now, here's what we find: we're very involved in business in China, and everyone in China is an entrepreneur. Sometimes, you can almost feel at home. Everyone wants to start a business, but they're stronger on the desire to start a business than they are on building innovation-based businesses. The issue of innovation in China is mostly grit, and I don't believe... And it should not be understood from me to be an insult to the Chinese people. It's a fact. It's a different culture. And within their culture, there is a greater tradition of listening, of acting respectfully, of inculcating the received knowledge of your elders. So, we have this tremendous number of Chinese who really are driven to do things in business, but there's not a great deal of innovation. This shows up in research in China, and it shows up with companies in China. Now, this also marks phenomenal opportunity between China and Israel. There's been billions of dollars of investment from Chinese companies into Israeli companies as well as the acquisition of Israeli companies by Chinese companies. And it's brilliant, because what are we good at? We're great at inventing. We're good at developing, but we're certainly not a place for low-cost manufacturing, and we're a really, really small market. So, the opportunities between Chinese businesses and Israeli businesses is just fantastic. We just fit with each other in so many ways. Now, that's not to say it's easy. There are big cultural differences as we've just discussed and many challenges, but the opportunity is fantastic; this is what makes us a match because what they're really, good at, and what we are really, really good at are two different things. And that's says opportunity for partnership."

"That's a terrific way of looking at it. Are there any other countries that come to mind, that have any similarities at all?"

"Well, it's very interesting because we spend a lot of time traveling and talking to business associates in a variety of countries. Let me contrast Israel with another Asian country---Singapore. In 2015, we went public in Singapore, and in 2016, we established Trendlines Medical Singapore as our new incubator and the center for our medical device investments in Singapore and the region. The Republic of Singapore's total population is 5.5 million people. Incredibly successful. And what we see there are some really, strong business people who truly understand, in a most profound way, business and finance issues. But because the country is so successful, I would suggest, there is a smaller number of entrepreneurs than you would want to find there. On the other hand, there's inventions, very fine universities, tremendous respect for education. Yet, they suffer from a lack of entrepreneurs because the country is so successful." At the time I am writing this, Trendlines had raised almost $10 million on the Singapore Stock Exchange.

"So, they're not as motivated to take chances?" I asked.

"The question becomes, why would you take that risk to be an entrepreneur when you've got a very nice job? In Singapore if you decide to quit your job this morning, you can have a new job in the afternoon. Unemployment in Singapore, especially for an educated individual, is half that of the States or Israel – effectively, no unemployment. There are certain structural differences in their economy which are fascinating. The only one I'll mention right now is that working for government is a very good job in Singapore, not because it's a job for lazy people to go hide, but because their government wants the best people and pays them very well. Lots of smart people who work extremely hard. So, government is one of the sectors in Singapore that has the best of people. I've never seen it anywhere else in the world. I certainly don't see it in America, and honestly, I don't see it in Israel. Government does not suck up the best of people. Certainly, there are many good exceptions, but in a general sense, you'll find a very high percentage of very smart, very driven people in the Singapore government."

"Not the average bureaucrat. You get people that are highly qualified and motivated, which is really unique."

"That's very well said. And an effective way to think of it. The average bureaucrat in America, versus the average, and I'll use the word 'bureaucrat' again in Singapore. These are two incredibly different people."

"And in terms of expediting innovation, what I find quite often is that, especially here in the States, but in many other places too, that people just look at it as a giant morass that they can't navigate, as in, 'That's the government.' It's like saying, 'That's corporate.' And I don't see that same sense in Israel at all. There are ways to maneuver in the systems and try to get things done."

"A great way to think of it is, someone expressed to me once, when you're looking at various governments, ask, are they producing red tape or are they rolling out red carpet? And we certainly see tremendous differences on that in various places. In Israel, as part of that entrepreneurial culture, as part of the inability to accept the word no, Israelis will learn how to get something done even if it's against the rules. And the army teaches that as well because the army is very mission-oriented. You're not waiting for your commander to give you an order. You understand what the mission is, and it's your responsibility to achieve it even if you lose your commander during the battle."

"You sound like you have personal experience that has informed what you see as the role of the military in the government and innovation."

"I served sometime in the Israeli military and all three of my daughters have been through the army, so you don't live in Israel without having an army experience from your friends, from your family, and very often, from yourself."

"So, you have the mission-based aspect of the army, the connections that people might have established in the army, the innovative aspect of Israeli army high-tech/bio-tech, and the leadership training of the army. Companies try to recruit the top people from the army, right? So, you all do the same thing?"

"All of us are looking to invest in the same kind of people. For Trendlines, it's a major focus. We're all looking and we all want to be involved with people who are really dedicated, who are passionate, who are driven. Those are the most important things to us. In interviews, I look for that – we always evaluate people and markets before we focus on technology. The army helps us because the Army helps shape people into what we're looking for. So, when we invest, we're looking, first, at people. Secondly, we're looking at markets. We really, really need focus in our investing. We want to understand what's the market need, and then it's how do you fill it. That's the critical approach for us. It's people, market need, and then the technology," Dollinger said.

"Right. So, number one is looking at dedicated, driven, passionate people. Number two, the market. And number three, the technology?"

"You bet. If there's a problem with the technology, there's a reasonable chance we can fix it. We're a country filled with a lot of smart engineers, a lot of smart people. If we make a mistake about the market, well, maybe we can pivot, maybe we can make that change to adjust to what was misunderstood, or what changed. But when it comes to people...I studied psychology, but they didn't teach me how to fix someone. So, we really need to get it right with people."

"So, what about the vetting process? How formal is your screening?"

"At Trendlines we very slowly make an initial investment. We're wholly focused on doing everything as fast as possible, except for that. From the time that our staff meet you, and we start to talk about your invention, and we make that investment, start a company together, it can be nine months, and we like that process because we want to get to know you. We want to understand your thinking, we want to know, 'Can we be comfortable together?' because we're going to be living together for a few years. You're in our offices for at least two to three years and you're working with all of our staff."

6

MEDICAL MARIJUANA

I spoke to Dr. Raphael Mechoulam, an Israeli organic chemist and professor of Medicinal Chemistry and Natural Products at Hebrew University Hadassah Medical School and School of Pharmacy, Institute for Drug Research. He is best known for his work (together with Y. Gaoni) in the isolation, structure elucidation and total synthesis of Δ9-tetrahydrocannabinol, the main active principle of cannabis and for the isolation and the identification of the endogenous cannabinoids. Dr. Mechoulam has received many honors including honorary doctorates from Spain and USA, the Israel Prize in 2000, the European College of Neuropsychopharmacology

Lifetime Achievement Award in 2006 and the Rothschild Prize in 2016.

While working at the Weizmann Institute of Science in Rehovot, Mechoulam secured hashish from the head of Israel's investigative branch of the national police for use in his studies, and in 1963 his research group determined the structure of CBD (cannabidiol). By 1964 they had isolated and synthesized THC (tetrahydrocannabinol), the main psychoactive compound of cannabis. Over the years he has continued to research the chemistry of endogenous cannabinoids and synthesis of novel compounds to be tested as drugs against pain, epilepsy, inflammation, high blood pressure and cancer. He received a grant from the US National Institutes of Health and has collaborated with colleagues from all over the world.

"How did you get started with all this?" I asked.

"We started working on cannabis, I started working in the early 60's. I was a young man then," Mechoulam said. "This whole field has undergone basically three major phases. The first phase was elucidating the chemistry of cannabis. Today modern science cannot be done if the chemistry is not there. Pharmacology cannot do mixtures, or mixtures that are not well-defined. We started with chemistry, and surprisingly the chemistry of cannabis was not well-known at that time. Morphine had been isolated from opium almost 130 years previously, and cocaine had been isolated from coca leaves 100 years previously, but surprisingly the cannabis chemistry was not known, and each pharmacology was kind of vague, and there were no real clinical trials."

"What next?" I asked.

"We started with the chemistry, and we isolated what I believe is for the first time THC, the active component. At that time, it was not known if there was one compound or numerous compounds. Well, it turned out that it is essentially the only active compound. Although its activity can be affected by additional constituents. This is something we called the entourage effect. We then isolate about half a dozen compounds, and elucidated their structures, and this has been going on now for 50 years by many groups in the States and many other places. There are about 80 compounds of the same type known, but the only one that's psychoactive to any significant extent/substantial/considerable extent is THC, which we isolated in 1964."

"What other compounds caught your attention?" I asked.

"Another compound which is of major interest is cannabidiol. We elucidated its structure in 1963, and then we worked on, besides on the chemistry, the metabolism and pharmacology for quite some years. The one major thing that was not known about THC for many years was the mechanism. How does THC work? It turns out that there are two receptors. The first one discovered by Allyn Howlett in the States. Receptors don't exist because there is a compound out there in a plant, they exist because we make compounds, neurotransmitters in this case. We went ahead trying to find out these neurotransmitters. This is the second phase of cannabinoid research, working on the endogenous compounds that we make, not the plant, we make them. Our brain makes them, our body makes them."

"And what did you look at next?" I asked.

"In the 90's we identified two compounds that bind to the cannabinoid receptors," Mechoulam said. "It took quite a lot of work. One we called anandamide, and the other is 2AG. These two compounds are essentially the major endogenous neurotransmitters of the cannabinoid system. There are thousands and thousands of papers on these two compounds."

"I researched and found that in the 1990's you, William Devane, Lumir Hanus and Aviva Breuer identified and synthesized the first endogenous cannabinoid in the human brain. Roger Pertwee in the UK compared its activity with that of THC and found almost parallel activity. You named it anandamide, the Sanskrit word for "supreme joy" or "bliss." Two years later you discovered the endogenous compound 2-AG. What other neurotransmitters have you worked on?" I asked.

"There is now a whole neurotransmitter system based on these two receptors CB1 and CB2. One of them, known as CB1, is found in larger amounts than any other receptor. So, people have been looking at the system of the receptors, endogenous cannabinoids, the enzymes that form and that break them down. So, there is a huge amount of work, and recently researchers at NIH published a review saying endocannabinoids are involved in essentially all human diseases. It's a rather strong statement, but it seems to be almost certainly true. This is the second stage, and quite a lot of work has been going on."

"And now?"

"Now we are at the third stage, I believe we can call that a third stage. Anandamide is a compound formed from fatty acid bound to an amino acid derivative. But it turns out there are about 200 compounds of the same type in our body, most of them in the brain. It turns out that all these compounds, or at least those that have been investigated, are of extreme physiological importance. One of them, or several of them, cause vasodilation, which is important after brain injury. There's another one which we found that is involved of osteoporosis, women's osteoporosis. There is quite a lot of interest in all these compounds, and quite a few people are working on them. There is work on all three phases of cannabinoids. You see, anandamide is a compound which

THC mimics its actions. By chance, THC binds to the same receptors where the anandamides bind. Both the anandamide and 2AG, the twin, and the cannabinoid are of major importance. (Erased, written anew) – Anandamide is made of a fatty acid, arachidonic acid, bound to a derivative of amino acid, ethanolamide. There are lots of chemical possibilities, and the body has learned, apparently, to make related compounds of additional fatty acids, long chain fatty acids, oleic acid, palmitic acid, stearic acid. All kinds of acids in our bodies that bind to amino acids or derivatives of amino acids."

"How do they work to help us?" I asked.

"It turns out that the body is saving energy by using the same system to produce additional compounds of the same type, and many of these compounds are pretty active. Some of them are made in the brain after a brain injury. Prof Esther Shohami and I have published quite a bit on showing that after brain injury in a mouse the brain starts producing compounds of this type, and they lower the damage. If we take compounds of this type, and we have done that with several of these, and we give to the mice after injury, then the damage is lower. These compounds are the endogenous protectors of what's going on in the brain after damage, so that's one thing that these compounds do."

The endocannabinoid system is a ubiquitous lipid signaling system that we now know appeared early in evolution and has important regulatory functions throughout the body in all vertebrates. It consists of a family of G-protein-coupled receptors, the cannabinoid receptors (CB1 found in the brain and many peripheral tissues, and CB2, primarily found in immune cells); endoligands to activate these receptors; and two enzymes, the fatty acid amide hydrolase and the monoacylglycerol lipase, to metabolize the endoligands. The endoligands of the cannabinoid receptor system, small molecules derived from arachidonic acid, are called endocannabinoids.

Cannabinoid receptors (primarily CB1) are found in higher concentrations than any other receptor in the brain. are densely distributed in both neuronal and glial areas, and the endocannabinoids are thought to play a critical neuromodulatory role. Cannabinoid CB1 receptor activation is known to modify the release of several neurotransmitters, including glutamate and gamma-aminobutyric acid, and to be involved in motor control, cognition, memory consolidation, emotional responses, motivated behavior and homeostasis.

"What else?" I asked.

"Often research starts out with the assumption that it has nothing to do with cannabinoids, and then it turns out that it has to do with cannabinoids. It was shown many years ago that women in the Mediterranean region have much less osteoporosis than the women in the northern countries. It was believed it's due to olive oil, which is the only oil that's being consumed by women in this particular region. So, we looked at olive oil and its major constituent, and we found that a metabolite of the major constituent of olive oil is a compound that our body produces, and it is a very, very effective anti-osteoporosis agent. That's one of the reasons why many women with that diet do not have major osteoporosis, because they have prominent levels of this particular compound."

"Do you get that just from commercial olive oil that you would use on salads or in the Mediterranean diet? Is it the same type of olive oil?" I asked.

"This particular compound is the oleic acid bound to the amino acid serine. No, it is not in commercial olive oil. It is a metabolite of oleic acid, which is a major constituent of olive oil. Here we have another quite different type of activity, which we basically didn't expect. Now many people are looking at compounds of this type. One of these compounds that has been around for many years is palmitoylethanolamide, which is used in Europe as an anti-inflammatory compound, and it belongs to the same type of materials. I believe that the cannabinoid field has moved from preliminary stages/initial stages, and chances are that endocannabinoid-like compounds will be major drugs, hopefully for a variety of diseases," Mechoulam said.

"You have been quoted as saying, 'There is almost no physiological system that has been considered in which endocannabinoids don't play a certain part.'"

"True," Mechoulam said.

"In the United States and around the world we talk about organic and alternative and integrative therapy. We know that many medicines, such as the ones I use in dermatology every day, were plant-derived. Has this given you even more faith or interest in terms of deriving things from plant-based products?" I asked.

"Many of our drugs are modified natural products. Old antibiotics are natural products. We now mostly use modified products. You cannot buy penicillin in a pharmacy; you buy a derivative of penicillin. You cannot buy cortisone. You use a derivative of cortisone, which is probably better like Prednisone. A vast number of drugs are derivatives from natural products.

"Given the anti-inflammatory effects, is there any general correlation between cannabinoids and steroids? "I asked.

"One thing that ties the two groups together is that both are lipid-soluble compounds. The steroids and cannabinoids, whether they're plant cannabinoids or endogenous cannabinoids, they're all lipid-soluble. There seems to be something common going on there, but we don't know enough about it," Mechoulam said.

"On a personal basis, reading about your history, you

came from a medical family. Your father was a physician?"

"Yes, he was. And two of my daughters are physicians."

"And your mother?"

"My mother studied in Berlin for a year or two, but she came back, and was a housewife. At that time, most women didn't go out and work, they stayed mostly at home."

"How did your family background motivate you to consider the research you're doing, or did it?"

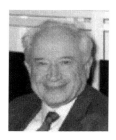

Dr. Raphael Mechoulam

"I started as an organic chemist, and my Ph. D. thesis was in organic chemistry, but in a field that is closely related to medicine. Steroids, as a matter of a fact. I was doing extensive research on steroids, and I found that working between chemistry and physiology is exciting. I've been working on natural products ever since, both in the chemistry and pharmacology. We've done quite a lot of clinical trials on cannabinoids. This is one thing that we don't know enough about. There have been very few clinical trials for several reasons, probably political mostly. For example, in cancer, hundreds of thousands of people use cannabinoids in cancer. There hasn't been a single modern clinical trial with any cancer with cannabinoids."

"What type of trials?" I asked.

"We did a clinical trial with epilepsy using cannabidiol, and that was done 35 years ago. We published this small trial on 15 patients with pure cannabidiol. They got high doses of cannabidiol, and the patients, all of them, had epilepsy that was not being helped by their existing drugs. It helped. We had eight placebo patients, seven that got the drug, and four out of the seven did not have any attacks while they're being treated with prominent levels/elevated levels of cannabidiol. The other three had much less. So, I thought that neurologists would go ahead and expand this small clinical trial – it obviously was important. Surprisingly nothing happened for about 35 years. Then parents of children that have epilepsy realized that cannabidiol may help and started using cannabis with elevated levels of cannabidiol. In many cases it worked. A major clinical trial is being done now in the US. It should have been done 30 years previously. It's a shame. The same is true for schizophrenia; A major clinical group in Germany found a few years ago that cannabidiol is pretty good in schizophrenia without having any side effects. But yet, it is not being developed as a drug." Mechoulam said.

"What about in dementia?" I asked.

"I'm also interested in Alzheimer's. Cannabinoids seem to affect Alzheimer's. Numerous groups have shown that that cannabinoids block some of the effects of Alzheimer's."

"What about in dermatology?" I asked.

"We need more clinical trials to learn and research in humans. But speaking of your own field, cannabidiol has been shown by a very good by an Italian group to cause methylation of DNA, and to change actually the basis of some diseases, including in skin disease such as psoriasis. They found that cannabidiol was pretty useful by binding with DNA and blocking down the production of undesirable compounds. So apparently, cannabidiol, which has a lot of activities, acts by, in part at least, through an epigenetic pathway, namely methylating DNA that works overtime. That's one of the ways that it blocks undesirable activity."

"Fascinating," I said.

"If this is a general phenomenon or not we don't know yet. There have been very few papers on that, but it seems we have a drug that acts not only on the symptoms but also the disease. Because the basis of a disease in many cases may be over activity of DNA."

"Within somebody's own lifetime it could change the disease structure itself rather than being passed on…"

"Yes. It can change temporarily at least, the activity of DNA. It was published by a group in Italy, led by Mauro Maccarrone."

"What is the newest research about?" I asked.

"There are quite a few companies, including major ones, that are working on compounds that work on the CB2 receptor alone. The CB2 receptor does not cause psychoactivity, and therefore it's of importance. It's a defense mechanism of a sort, if you wish. A compound that acts on the CB2 receptor alone is of importance," Mechoulam said.

"How does it work?"

"Cannabidiol works through a different mechanism than THC, completely different. As a matter of fact, cannabidiol affects the activity of THC. When you speak of medical marijuana in the United States there is a problem because I'm not sure what medical marijuana is. It can have a little bit of THC, a lot of THC, little bit of this, little bit of that, and physicians do not like to work with compounds that are not well-defined. When you give a patient a drug you know exactly how much you're giving, how often he should take it, et cetera. Not just take something, bye bye. We are trying here in Israel to quantify the amount of material present in medical marijuana, so we shall have three or four types of medical marijuana, and they will be sold in drugstores and pharmacies, and they will have to indicate, at least at the beginning, the levels of THC, the levels of CBD, and the physicians and the pharmacists will know what kind of medical marijuana fits a certain disease. For epilepsy it's essentially pure CBD, for post-trauma it's mostly THC. Schizophrenia, mostly CBD."

"What is the status of marijuana in Israel now?"

"There is a department in the Ministry of Health which deals with cannabis. A person who thinks he needs cannabis or his physician thinks he needs cannabis, the physician can apply, not the sick person. The physician can apply to the Ministry, saying we've tried drug A, drug B, drug C, doesn't work; we want to see whether medical marijuana will work. So, the physician applies and the physicians at the Ministry of Health have to approve it. There are 27,000 patients now that have medical marijuana for a variety of diseases, mostly pain, cancers, (erased) gastrointestinal diseases. Not for skin diseases, to the best of my knowledge. But things change all the time."

"So, it's not that difficult for a needy patient to get, such as someone with severe pain and no previous relief?"

"No, it is not difficult. The physician must be a specialist. A pain specialist must/should apply for a medical cannabis for pain, neurologist for neurological diseases, and so on. It is not difficult if it's within the medical areas that have been approved. For additional areas, like asthma for example, one must look at the specific patients (erased). Medical cannabis works on asthma in some cases, not all."

"What about recreational use?" I asked.

"That is a different thing. Recreational use is illegal in Israel. I think there should be a complete separation between the two. The recreational thing is a social issue that must be approved, in a democratic country, by the entire public. It has to be agreed upon by a vote... Medical things have to be decided by the medical profession, by the scientists. That's the way it's going here. I believe that Israel is a rather conservative country, and if tomorrow morning there was a vote I think that most of the population will say no to legal recreational marijuana. But on the other hand, at present the police will not open a criminal file finding a 15-year old kid smoking cannabis for the first time. They'll make a little bit of fuss about it, but will not send him to trial."

"With the products that you're working with, the CBD and THC and so forth, it sounds like there's just a world of research and application possibilities both in affecting disease itself and in the understanding different disease etiologies that tie in with cannabinoids. All very helpful as long as there's more clinical trials," I said.

"You're right. But if we don't have clinical trials we have a major, major problem. It shouldn't be that way. That example I gave you with epilepsy, it's unbelievable that something that was published 35 years ago, it took so many years to go ahead. I think basically that there is a lot of promise, but it must be well-channeled and researched before it becomes used as approved major drugs.

"I see a tremendous amount of potential here, and you've been a pioneer in this. It's a pleasure and an honor to talk with you about all this. In one of the articles I read about you they called you the father of cannabis. Do you like that?" I asked.

"Well, probably the grandfather."

The world legal cannabis sales totaled $150 billion last year. In the United States alone the sales are expected to reach $21.8 billion by 2020. What is happening in marijuana research and development now in Israel?

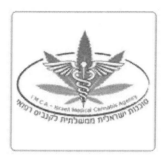

Medical Cannabis Uni, State of Israel, Ministry of Health

Israel is at the forefront of research and export due to technical, agricultural, and governmental policies overflowing with innovation. In January of 2017, the Israeli government invested $2.13 million in 13 cannabis research projects including MS, metabolic syndrome, preventing transplanted organ rejection, and inhibiting the development of harmful bacteria. Many new companies have sprouted up based on the initial efforts of Professor Mechoulam and other cannabinoid scientists along with the encouragement of cannabis research since the 1960s by Israel's government. In 2015, CNN medical correspondent Dr. Sanjay Gupta called Israel "the medical marijuana research capital."

Kalytera Therapeutics, Inc. is a clinical-stage pharmaceutical company developing cannabinoid prevention and therapeutics for Graft versus Host Disease ("GvHD"). The company is also developing a new class of proprietary CBD therapeutics and recently licensed two synthetic cannabis derivatives from the Hebrew University's technology transfer company Yissum. The derivatives are expected to have eventual use in treating osteoporosis, bone fractures and other diseases.

The Hebrew University of Jerusalem has a multidisciplinary center on cannabinoid research. And it appears that Professor Mechoulam's dreams of more clinical trials is becoming a reality. Israeli scientists are using their genetic engineering expertise to modify marijuana's molecular structure to target cannabinoids to specific receptors for treating diseases and symptoms. Hebrew University researchers have synthesized 22 versions of the cannabinoid THC for treating neurological, inflammatory, and other diseases.

ISA Scientific is an Israeli-American biopharmaceutical company that is testing the effects of CBD against diabetes as well as inflammatory and heart diseases. Although CBD can be obtained from marijuana, it is particularly abundant in hemp, a plant with no psychoactive properties and thus no potential for abuse. One of ISA Scientific's CBD production facilities is in China. Not only the world's largest hemp producer. China also represents an enormous potential/an immense potential market for the company's therapeutic products because the Chinese account for one-third of the approximately 371 million diabetics globally.

Tikun Olam is the first and foremost supplier of medical cannabis in Israel, and one of the leading medical cannabis companies in the world. The company is privately held and has been operating under license from the Israel Ministry of Health since 2007. According to its website, it has developed a range of proprietary varieties – perhaps up to 230 – used in clinical medical trials. Tikun Olam is a vertically integrated company – from plant to patient, and is founder of the first professional cannabis Nursing Clinic, located in Tel Aviv. "The patient takes the product for the first time under the supervision and guidance of a nurse. The counseling includes guidance of dosage, potential side effects, and fitting the suitable strains" based on the knowledge of the nurses to" adjust the treatment to the patient's medical condition, his weight and energy, his symptoms and their severity." In 2016 Tikun Olam expanded its business to the US and established a subsidiary company Tikun Olam USA (Tikun). The company invented a new varietal called Avidekel, which at 0% THC and 15.8% CBD provides all the healing and anti-inflammatory power of cannabidiol with no discernable high.

Although Professor Mechoulam noted Israel's conservative nature, in January 2017 the government announced plans to decriminalize personal marijuana use followed a month later by a government committee approving cannabis export. Reforms from 2016 opened licensing for as many marijuana growers as the market will support and over 200 individuals and groups have applied to join Israel's current eight cannabis farms.

7

DIGITAL HEALTH

I spoke with Stephen M. Shapiro, managing partner of eHealth Ventures, LLC, about his role in digital health.

"I was working in digital health, mainly in electronic health records, EMR space with a US company, interestingly we used Israeli technology," Shapiro said. "We contracted all the software to be developed in Israel. During that time, I learned a lot about healthcare in the Israeli market. More specifically how they use big data, Electronic Medical Records (EMR) and other digital technology to improve outcomes and lower costs. With my current work in Israel I understood how they're 10 years ahead of us, maybe more, in electronic health records, telemedicine and ways to use technology to improve health resulting in the cost of healthcare to be one third of the US, the life expectancy of an Israeli to be longer than the life expectancy of a US person, an Israeli has an encounter with a doctor more often than we do."

"Interesting, I can see why you wanted to get more involved. How did it happen? I asked"

"During my work in Israel in the Electronic Health Record (EHR) space I met and became friends with Talor Sax. Talor spent most of his career in this space, doing development for Maccabi Healthcare and others. There are four major HMOs in Israel with Maccabi Healthcare being the second largest, with over two million members. More on Maccabi later.

Talor explained to me about the incubator program in Israel and how Israel is becoming a world leader in "digital health" Talor asked me to join him in creating eHealth Ventures to take advantage of this opportunity. He said there were no incubators that were totally focused on digital health, and we recognized that digital health was growing rapidly. It may be the fastest growing sector in healthcare in the world today and it is just getting started"

"Tell me about your background before healthcare." I asked.

"I started in computers, or data processing as it was called back in the late 1960s to computerize accounting systems for businesses, which was innovative at that time," Shapiro said. "In the middle '80s, I'd entered the cellular phone industry when we probably had half-a-million users in the US, with a lot of skeptics saying there is no need for cellular phones. We proved the skeptics wrong. After a successful exit in the cellular phone industry I did consulting ending up in the EHR space in 2011. So, career-wise, maybe I'm at substantial risk/considerable risk. I get into things very early, and fortunately, they've panned out. Digital Health is proving to be disruptive to healthcare like computers were to businesses and cellular phones were to communications. There's such a need for it."

"What happened next?"

"Talor and I got together, and we put together a business plan and a strategy then we met with the leadership at Maccabi Healthcare to interest them to partner with us. They loved the idea and had enough confidence in Talor and I to partner with us. Our mission is to find, fund and grow early stage Israeli companies in digital health."

"Why Israel?" I asked.

"A strong technology base here, we like the digital health space opportunity, and under the Incubator Program, the government will put in 85% of the funding for a company while taking no equity. The government will only get their loan back if the company generates revenue. They take a small royalty until the loan is paid off in addition to a small interest charge. If the company fails the loan is forgiven allowing the entrepreneur to move forward in other areas. The advantage of this program for us as investors is we can put 15% of the money as equity in the portfolio company while allowing us to negotiate with the owner for the entire investment from the Government and from us. For each portfolio company, we will get from 20% to 49% equity. This provides a highly leveraged investment for our limited partners."

"What else have you done to succeed?" I asked.

"So that's one side of it. The second side of it, we created a platform for start-up companies to have a higher chance of success then most companies that fail at the early stage. We do it by creating a strong consortium that can add substantial value to our selection process as well as for the portfolio company once they enter our incubator. Our consortium or strategic partners include world-class healthcare organizations like The Cleveland Clinic, Amgen, Maccabi Healthcare and others. They add considerable value in three ways: 1: Assist in the due diligence process, 2: Help/Aid the portfolio companies while they are in the incubator and 3: Assist in commercialization. Here is more detail:

Our strategic partners help us in the due diligence process they help identify the right companies for the incubator. We look for companies that solve a problem, have technology that has the potential to be disruptive technology, and have a quantifiable revenue model. We have created a very specific, regimented process to assess companies. Once we see the company meets our basic qualifications we ask our healthcare partners to assist by looking at the technology and determine the need and where possible, clinically validate the technology. Once we get reviews from our healthcare partners we follow our due diligence process. This could take six months. We then have to must/should submit our findings to the Israel Innovation Authority. They perform a review, meet with our Israeli team and with the principals of the company being evaluated. Once approved by the Israel Innovation Authority we will complete our legal diligence and present to eHealth Ventures Investment committee. If approved they will become a portfolio company in our incubator."

"How about getting to market?" I asked.

"When they're ready to commercialize, we will utilize our consortium of international partners to help with the markets and commercialization. Israel's a very small consumer market. They are excellent in development of technology, but to commercialize and grow the company they must sell outside of Israel. We want and have the ecosystem to help each of these companies launch internationally."

"What is your major focus?"

"Software-related in the digital health space, we look at software that will help the physician, the specialist, and others to do their job better. A lot of it is to make healthcare more personal and accessible. We see telemedicine as one game changer. Another is personal health that allows the patient to take ownership of their own health. As you know daily new healthcare related apps and devices reach the market. It is critical that the data being collected on the individual provide to the clinician actionable information at the right time. We have limitless data collected on our personal devises, so this information needs to be analyzed identifying what is critical to the individual's health. AI and big data are being utilized. This is a complex area that we can go into later."

"I sometimes joke with my patients, although it's frustrating, that any day that ends with the letter 'y', we have to do your prior authorization. We have a big practice and we spend at least 40% of our time with prior authorizations, gathering previous lab, figuring out data, dealing with redundancy and inefficiency. We probably have fifteen patients per day where they came in from another provider, we had to call the providers or facilities, find out what their lab work was, see how that relates to what they have, do they have any history of diseases that has been verified, or any other issues. All this is just so time-consuming and I could focus on taking care of the patients, and we see this all day. It's endemic in our system."

"Oh, I totally agree," Shapiro said. "When I was in electronic health records, the EMR space, the doctors just hated the time it took to enter data into their EHR. I was in this early when 'meaningful use' was picking up, and the government was trying to force physicians to adapt to it. Many doctors I saw said they would either retire early, because they didn't want to deal with it, or they would sell their practice to a hospital. They would get out of their practice, because medicine to them was not what it was earlier in their careers."

"On a personal basis though, you just hit the nail on

the head, because I see it happening all the time with really good qualified physicians that have... really at the peak of their career as far as experience...so much frustration with it now that they just throw in the towel."

"I understand."

"Let me ask you a few questions and you choose where to start. By talking to various people, I've heard some consistencies in what people think is "The Israel Effect" in the medical startup nation. One of them has to do with innovation, another one has to do with Israel and the Jews, another has to do with the Army and the long-term connections there, and also the Russian Aliyah. What has set the scene for the remarkable success in Israeli medicine?"

"Let me first tie the success in with the Russian Aliyah. When all the Russians came to Israel, Israel recognized that they had a lot of new smart Israelis. So, the government created this incubator concept, where they could take this brain power and break them into different areas of interest. The Government separated them into rooms based on their expertise and let them solve problems and come up with companies or ideas, and that was the start of the Incubator Program."

"Please tell me more about the incubator program," I said.

"The government has a structured request for proposal (RFP) process when they decide to open a new incubator for interested groups to compete to get a license to own and operate an incubator. Israel is a world leader in "exits" of technology companies. The Incubator program has been a proven source for entrepreneurs to develop their technology and become an attraction for buyouts or mergers. This has resulted in a high level of interest by world-class companies to take part in the incubator program. One benefit of having this license is to enjoy the Government involvement. Maybe it sounds bureaucratic, but we value the assistance of the highly qualified team from the Israel Innovation Authority. They provide useful feedback during our selection process and of course the funding that I mentioned earlier the Government provides to the portfolio companies. Once you're granted the license, and believe me it was a long, competitive process you're given a license for eight years, and at the end of eight years, you can reapply. So, some of the people we compete with are experienced in the program since their eight years are up and they're reapplying, most had a very good track record. The Israel Government has done an excellent job to get the best world-class companies to compete to be granted this license. Goals of this program include creating jobs in Israel, stimulating innovation, and to help the economy grow. The focus is not just in healthcare, there are agriculture, water incubators, cyber-security incubators, biotech incubators, so it touches many, many different spaces. To help ensure success of a company, they will be funded in the incubator for two years, so that really gets them time to develop their business, create a strong go to market strategy, when they leave, they're ready to commercialize and to get their next round of funding. The incubator not only provides office space for the companies, but very specific help on setting up their business, budgeting, human resources, marketing, assistance with clinical trials, product development and much more."

"What about accelerators?" I asked.

"Yes, there are also lots of accelerators and new ones coming. Some of them are run by Microsoft and IBM as well as other International companies have accelerators in Israel with a goal to help these entrepreneurs create an idea to a company. When these companies are successful, the accelerator sponsor wants them to use their technology and products. Possibly the accelerator sponsor will one-day purchase the technology being developed. Most incubators look at the graduates of the accelerator program as a source of deal flow. These programs help fuel the Israeli economy. So, one side is the economic encouragement in Israel. The government does provide a lot of financial incentives. Next, the mentality they get in the military... there's two sides. The IDF takes them out of high school when they're still bright and things are forming in their brain, and they create a way of thinking, a way of challenging assumptions, out of the box, what to do in a crisis. So, they get them at an early age, and so that stays with them when they leave the military. If I fail, okay. I have to pick myself up and I have to learn from that failure, and how do I improve moving forward? In fact, probably most of the entrepreneurs I talk to, have had companies that have failed."

"That confirms what I have heard many times," I said.

"And so, the culture kind of accepts it and people accept it. It's not that failure is good, but there are lessons to learn from failure. It doesn't mean you're a loser by failing; it could be the reverse. And I think they get that critical thinking from the military. Another thing they get out of the military is that the military uses advanced technology, and there are a lot of examples of things that were thought of in the military. In fact, we're talking to one company that has a phone app that will look at a person's skin to help detect a cancerous lesion that they claim they are using technology that started in the military. Consistently we've seen cases where companies take technology that was originally used for a different purpose and now used in medicine."

"And what about the Israeli culture?" I asked.

"I meet a lot with entrepreneurs. I probably have met with 100 since we started. We clearly see the confidence, drive and spirit that they have. It's something about that environment that I have not seen anywhere else in the world, that people...they want to start out, they want to create something. I think it's a great, great mentality they have. Now it can go both ways. Some of them think they have the answers to everything, and they're not coachable, and that's a key trait when you look at an individual. Is that person coachable? And many of them are not coachable."

"But the ones that are coachable have a good country to work in?"

"Yes. A big part is the environment in Israel. Israel is very small and has limited resources, so they must learn to do more with less. I think if you invest money in a company, a fear is they're going to blow through that money fast so how do they use the money? Part of the Israeli culture is to appreciate what you have, learn to do more with less. Most Israelis know what it is to sacrifice and to come up creatively with ways to spend less money to accomplish the same thing. I think that's a big, big part of the success, with the limited resources, how an early stage company can go to the next level."

"You work in the US and Israel. What has been part

of your success?"

"Our first win was to get Maccabi Healthcare as a partner. Next was The Cleveland Clinic, who is also a great partner of ours that gives us a lot of credibility in Israel, because so many Israelis want to do business in the US. But it's not just the US. The whole Chinese phenomena in Israel is incredible, and one of our major investors is from China. Israel has become a gateway to the world. Their location, track record with technology, the arts and much more has created success to ease the flow of goods and services to the US, Europe, Asia and Africa."

"What about the Jewish factor, of our culture and learning, of questioning, all these factors that makes for a successful venture in entrepreneur?" I asked.

"I think about this point a lot. It's not so much the 'religious' factor, but the Jewish cultural factor. What percent of Israelis are secular Jews? The majority. Why? If you live in the United States, in a country where you're a minority, you tend to belong to a Jewish organization, a synagogue, just to be around fellow Jews, and that's why where you belong. If you're in Israel, Jewishness is everywhere. Several years ago, my wife and I were in Israel during Hanukah. We would see public menorahs everywhere. Like one would see Christmas Trees in the US. One of my favorite stories in Israel was on the last night of Hanukah, which happen to be on Sunday night. We wanted to watch NFL football so we went to a sports bar to watch a one o'clock football game, which is at night in Israel. The bartender lit a Hanukah menorah that was sitting on the bar; everybody did the blessings and sang Hanukah songs. Where else would that happen?"

"What I've heard consistently from people is that, 'China's has tremendous infrastructure but almost a stifling hierarchy, whereas Israel has very little hierarchy and infrastructure and an incredible entrepreneurship mentality.' So that's why it's a good match between the two because Israelis are able to move things along quicker than China does."

"Right. Being a small country does have some advantages, even in healthcare. If you get into an accident in Beersheba, and you live in Haifa, the attending clinician has immediately access to your health records. But that's part of their success; they learn and can act to not duplicate mistakes. The ecosystem that just builds on itself, which you cannot have in a country like the US, where there's too many darn jurisdictions. I looked at some software once, developed in Israel and used in Israel. If you dial 911 on your phone in Israel, the cellular phone video goes on, so the operator answering the 911 call can see where you are and what's happening, instantly."

"One of the main things I've been asking people about consistently is innovation, and you brought up some very good points. So, what is your goal, what do you personally hope to accomplish?"

"We have three goals for putting so much in to eHealth Ventures. First to help in the most meaningful way Israel and its people. Second to do what we can to improve healthcare delivery and last to make a little 'gelt' money. Thank you!"

Talor Sax is the CEO of eHealth Ventures.

"Please tell me about Israel and digital health," I asked.

"Let's go back in time. There was already a high-tech industry in Israel that started in the '70s. Intel and IBM and the big guys started to work here. And healthcare in general around the world was very low tech. Israel, because of the structure of the healthcare market and the use of HMOs, was ahead of the curve. Especially since 1991, with a new health law that came into effect in Israel, the HMOs had to become what is now known in the US as an accountable care organization. The main providers, the HMOs, had to become accountable for the expenses because they were getting paid per capita on a formulation that depended on age and health status. One of the main methods of accountability was the use of technology. The HMO today in Israel can show you real data of the entire medical record since 1991. And having this data and this infrastructure allows a much greater service. It was natural to us in Israel to adopt technology into healthcare. I started developing healthcare IT solutions in Israel back in 2001. I didn't know what was going on in the outside world," Sax said, laughing. "I had no idea. I was sure that we were doing what everybody else was doing. We opened the window and looked around us, and saw what had happened. That was when I understood that we are doing something special and that we should go outside and give this technology to the world. That is when I started to work outside of Israel," Sax said.

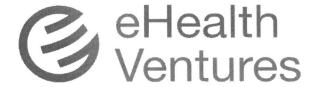

"After you looked and figured it out, what was the next step you made to connect to the outside world?"

"We visited to the US, to the Cleveland area. Later there were deals that we pursued in different places around the world, including Europe and the US mostly, but also India and Africa."

"So, the Israeli market structure was quite relevant?" I asked.

"Yes. It allowed us or forced the industry to computerize; having that alongside with the start-up nation spirit that was already there – the result was inevitable. The HMOs had a big part in technology use compared to the hospitals. HMOs are mostly about community care and Israel became highly advanced in technology in all of the HMOs. The general hospitals were computerized in terms of an EMR just in recent years. But the community side has been computerized for more than 20 years. HMOs in Israel are the main entities because they are not only the providers, they are also the payers. They play both roles, and it makes them very significant in the market," Sax said.

"Right. Did you have many people you knew from the army that are now important for your business?"

"Yes. The best example is that I'm working with Dr. Joseph Rosenblum. He's a Maccabi physician and serves as Chief Medical Officer at eHealth Ventures. In Maccabi, his formal role is Chief of Medical Informatics. Dr. Rosenblum was one of the founders of the computerized system in the army. He was there to build it from the beginning, years ago. "

"What has been the biggest challenge working

between Israel and the United States on a personal or professional basis?"

"There's a huge difference in culture," Sax said. "Our doctors use the same names of medications and procedures but the system and the culture of the system is completely different. It took me two years working in the US in the healthcare industry to fully understand how different it is. Our model here is closer to Europe than it is to the US and that is the main challenge that I've witnessed. I think that is what almost every young entrepreneur has faced. You can never assume that anything that works here would work anywhere else in the world in terms of medical technology. A device will work, but can you sell it in the same way? Is it the same entity that will make the decision of purchasing it? How will it all work? It's completely different."

"We certainly have a quagmire for getting things done here and the FDA often hinders us. In Israel, more people know each other and it's smaller, and you can avoid some of the problems that you can't avoid in the United States," I said.

"Yes, and I think the business opportunity for Israel entrepreneurs in 10 years, or even in five years, may not necessarily be in the US. I think there's a greater chance that China will become more and more of an actual market as well as Europe and maybe India over the US, and for several reasons. One reason is that the US is now quite saturated in most areas and the systems in the US are a lot different than in most other countries. I see more and more entrepreneurs and technologies that I would recommend go to Europe or China rather than go to the US. In the US you may find a market that you cannot penetrate because the big players are already there or the cost is so much higher that you can never raise enough money to get into it. Obviously, this is not a fact that is true for everybody, but I think there will be more and more of an opportunity in Europe, China and India for Israeli companies. We send delegations over, and we get a lot of delegations that are coming in. We have a Chinese delegation visiting our incubator at least once a month."

"Can you give me an example about China?" I asked.

"I took a guest from China to see a clinic at Maccabi

and to see the radiology system I built 10 years ago. The radiology information system works with 15 or 20 different locations in Israel where you can take the X-ray and then instead of printing it on film, it goes electronically to a center, where they have radiology interpreted and you get back the result within 20 minutes. Very effective but very common today. Perhaps it was less common 10 years ago when we launched it. And the Chinese man looked at me when we showed it to him and said, 'Wow, now I understand. We have the same equipment in China, the same machines, but we never figured out the way to write the software to do this.' And I can tell you that the cost of the software was ridiculously low, like $50,000-$70,000 to write for the entire system. They were overwhelmed, and I'm talking about six months ago. On the other hand, we see China making huge leaps in modernization of the health system and the willingness to adopt new digital solutions. This is why I see a big opportunity there."

"Amazing," I said.

"We created a software that streamlines everything and makes it so much more efficient. All the infrastructure is there. They come to Israel because they understand that we have the innovation they miss. What happened with this guy is because he learned what's going on in Israel and how the government is helping startups to evolve and how innovation is running, he's trying to do this in Shanghai right now."

"So, you keep up with him?"

"Yes, we keep in touch," Sax said. "He's moving very, very fast. He brought, after that, a group of his local government people to see how innovation works here so they can give him a budget. They are really fast to copy from us ideas and approaches. I asked another Chinese, one who is investing with us, 'What's going on there? Why are the Chinese all over us? What's happening?' And he said two interesting things. One thing is that there's a five-year plan in China and healthcare technology is one of the main goals for this five years. The plan sites Israel as a source for innovation and that is why we see so many incoming requests and visits from China to Israel. And secondly, I asked him, why do you invest so much in Israeli companies, not so much in American companies? He said he thinks that many Chinese see the US as an economic enemy, which is not the case with Israel, and therefore they are more comfortable cooperating with Israelis. But that's his idea. I don't know if it represents a lot of people in China."

"One of the items that I've gotten feedback on during almost every interview is the Russian Aliyah and its effect," I said. "Do you see Russia as robust a trade partner as China?"

"I had a visit in Russia in 2010 and I brought a delegation of their healthcare ministries to Israel to see our technology here," Sax said. "They're putting some effort and money into it, but the amount of money that they're putting in is ridiculous compared to western standards. I visited some public hospitals. I was overwhelmed with how poor and backward it is. But then you go to Moscow and see a private hospital. From the inside it was like any other modern hospital. So, as a system, I think they have a long way to go to stabilize the economy there before they can become a real significant trade partner that adopts technology and healthcare. But there's still opportunities there."

"So, what's next in digital health?" I asked.

"Pharmaceutical companies in general are now moving towards digital health. They understand that they need to go there and that business is becoming more than just selling the pills. A lot of international companies are building innovation centers in Israel or putting people on the ground in Israel, rather than any other countries, to focus on digital health. And that includes big companies like Novartis, Pfizer, and others that want to expand in Israel. Still, I think they are not always asking the right questions on how to utilize the new digital health technology."

I had an informative interview with Mr. Daniel A. Blumenthal, who served as the Deputy Consul for Economic Affairs at the Government of Israel Economic Mission to the Midwest in Chicago until 2016. There, he worked with Israeli companies who were interested in conducting business abroad. In the US there are five similar offices which support Israeli companies looking at the US as a market for their products or for research and development (R&D) partners or investments. "We help the Israeli company look for ways to engage with the market here in the US and help to develop and promote the product. In the healthcare field, Israeli companies write to us seeking assistance in many ways; finding doctors to evaluate a product, investment, understanding the FDA, and finding sites for clinical trials," he said. "Most aspects of doing business is the same in Israel as it is in the US, but there are also major differences that if not addressed will lead the company to a dead end. In healthcare, for instance, without understanding the US insurance industry and how reimbursement works, your idea, as amazing as it might be, isn't going anywhere." In addition to the US offices, the Israeli government runs 40 similar offices around the world.

Blumenthal stated, "The market in Israel is small, so it is often necessary for Israeli companies to expand into the rest of the world, often much earlier than you'd see most companies working abroad. In the US, we connect Israelis with experts in various fields who can shed light on the market needs and trends, ideas for further R&D and make introductions to institutions which can conduct clinical trials and pilot studies. Although many Israeli companies approach us with an idea or technology which has been tested in the Israeli market, until its proven in the US it's difficult to make much headway here. Luckily for Israelis, more and more Americans know about Israel's tech scene and beyond being Israel's largest trading partner, the US is also a huge source for joint development and investment activity. US companies and executives are increasingly engaged with what's happening in Israel and many are eager to find the right opportunities to get involved. That may start with a small pilot and it may grow to an acquisition and even a new office based in Israel – the path companies like Google, IBM, Medtronic, J&J, among many others, have followed.

Blumenthal continued, "As far as the output of Israel, although our office supports a variety of Israeli industries, our office has a heavy tech focus: about 90% of our work is with early stage technology companies. Israel has about 5,000 such companies, with close to 25% in healthcare. About 60% of those are considered medical device, where Israel has traditionally excelled; the rest are digital health, which is a rapidly growing field in Israel and worldwide, and to a lesser extent pharmaceutical which have a much longer and more expensive path to market."

"What makes Israel so unique?" I asked.

"Many factors contribute to Israel's successful technology scene. One thing our office focuses on which makes Israel unique is the government support system, largely managed by the Chief Scientist Office within the Ministry of Economy in Israel which has a budget of about $400 million to invest in Israeli companies. The idea is not to invest like a venture capital firm, but to leverage the investment with partnerships. Many years ago, the Government established "incubators" to support companies with various resources to encourage growth, but these incubators are different than what we know in the US; in Israel, incubators are government funded and privately operated. Usually there are multiple partners that come together to run them. You often see a multinational company alongside venture capital firms who together operate the incubator – selecting the companies and working with them on a regular basis - but receive the initial funding from the government. This allows more opportunities for the Israeli companies to reach their market and garner more investment down the line. The Chief Scientist Office funds the incubators with an initial investment of about 80%, and in that way the Israeli government encourages a multinational company to be partners and active in Israel. The government wants Israelis to look around the world for help, and as we've watched the Israel economy expand with technologies and partnerships so prevalent and the now well-known moniker "Startup Nation" adopted worldwide, it's worked."

As of Summer, 2016, Blumenthal's role in Chicago now focuses on one Israeli company's growth in the US market as he left his position with the Government of Israel to become the first employee and head U.S. operations for MDClone, an Israeli digital healthcare startup which launched in early 2016. MDClone was founded by the founders of Israel's most successful healthcare IT company, dbMotion, a healthcare data interoperability company, which was sold in 2013 to Chicago-based Allscripts for $235 million.

dbMotion is a fascinating story, growing from a small team with an idea to use the internet (a new concept back in the mid-1990s) as a way to share data across multiple healthcare settings without having to store the data at each site. Within a short period, the technology began to power universal access to healthcare records in Israel, meaning that for any patient, regardless of which doctor, which hospital, which part of the country or which insurance provider is being used, the patient's record is accessible to the care provider. This made Israel the first country in the world to have a fully connected healthcare system, something the US still struggles with mightily today. dbMotion found itself with an impressive product ahead of the market, as the US and the government was just starting to use the word "interoperability" in the mid-2000s. After much success in Israel, the company, then still a small operation in Israel, competed against some US technology giants for a project to connect electronic health systems at the University of Pittsburgh Medical Center (UPMC), one of the leading US medical centers, and won the project. That partnership grew to include an investment from UPMC and within a few years dbMotion was up and running as a company in Pittsburgh (along with its office back in Israel), with installations in hundreds of sites in the US. Ultimately, it was bought by Allscripts which still operates dbMotion and a team in Israel under its umbrella.

As is the case with many Israeli founders, there was still more innovation in the works. With more than 20 years in the healthcare data field, the founders were still baffled at how cumbersome the process was to obtain healthcare data for analysis and research. With billions on billions of dollars spent putting data into machines, the value of that investment remains incredibly limited. MDClone was launched in 2016 to address this challenge, and make it possible for fast retrieval of data by anyone interested in conducting an analysis. Its platform builds off the team's long history in the field and organizes healthcare data in such a way that anyone, even without programming skills or other specific medical knowledge, can ask a question and receive a data file ready for statistical analysis in minutes (something which typically takes months in today's world, even for seemingly straightforward medical questions). From there, however, MDClone's secret sauce is the way it protects patient privacy, as most people are not allowed to see real patient data because of regulations in place to protect patients. MDClone developed the only "zero-risk" solution on the market with an engine that produces "synthetic data," maintaining the statistical story of the real (identifiable) data but containing no real patient data – meaning it is impossible to identify a patient using MDClone's synthetic data. In this way, the data can be shared more freely and without lengthy legal barriers which prevent so much analysis from taking place. The data owners (hospitals, insurance companies and the like) still maintain control over the data in their systems and can decide to whom they want to provide access, including researchers, business analysts, and partners at external companies and institutions.

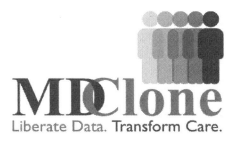

In a short time, MDClone has become one of the hottest healthcare startups in Israel, installing its platform throughout Israel at giants like Clalit and Maccabi (the two largest HMOs in Israel) along most of the largest hospitals including Assuta, Rambam, and Sheba. As of late 2017, Blumenthal and the team are beginning the expansion into the US with a number of pilot projects launching.

How do you efficiently and clearly convey important medical information to providers and patients?

I spoke with Rami Cohen, the Founder and CEO of Telesofia, a company founded in 2011 by a team of medical doctors and Internet industry veterans. Cohen holds a medical doctor degree from the Tel Aviv University and worked at the Vascular Surgery department in Tel-Aviv Sourasky (Ichilov) Medical Center and Assaf Harofeh Medical Center. Since 2001 Cohen helped several companies and start-ups with product development, launching and marketing in the online world.

Cohen and I had a very enjoyable conversation and I noted he is very passionate about his work. He and I discussed how a vast majority of people do not understand medical instructions from doctors and pharmacists. Others find hospital discharge orders confusing and new US regulations penalize hospitals for avoidable readmissions. Many have just been given a disease diagnosis and cannot wrap their minds around any even moderately complex instructions. Perhaps the most problematic is that thousands of patients daily seek emergency care due to an error in taking their medications.

Cohen's prescription? He combines the patient's digital medical record with a huge data library from thousands of pharmaceuticals and other sources to make a video that is produced automatically. The goal of Telesofia is to make medical information clear by providing patient education and engagement with personalized patient videos, accessible on any device. As per their website, "Telesofia Medical's proprietary platform allows healthcare providers to automatically generate branded personalized educational videos for patients based on their demographics, lab results, specific medical instructions, specific product used, and more. Each video is tailored to the specific patient, directed to low literacy level, and available on devices with no need to install a specific application or codec."

What is included in Telesofia's platform? The wide variety of applications include explaining proper use of medications, preparations for medical procedures, and providing discharge instructions. Each video is easily integrated into existing workflows and platforms, fully branded videos are sent to patients through text or email messages, or embedded in patient portals/apps. Telesofia has an R&D center in Tel Aviv and a business office in the United States, its main target market.

I spoke with Dr. Joseph Rosenblum, physician and Chief of Medical Informatics for Maccabi health.

"I began working in medical informatics in 1984," he said. "I started working in the Sheba Medical Center, which is the largest general-purpose hospital in Israel. I established at Sheba clinical computing, that practically didn't exist. I was in charge."

The Chaim Sheba Medical Center at Tel HaShomer was founded in 1948 and is affiliated with Tel Aviv University. It is located in the Tel HaShomer neighborhood of Ramat Gan, in the Tel Aviv District, and is the largest hospital in Israel, with 1700 beds.

"I established clinical computing," Rosenblum said. "I also did medical informatics in the IDF. As a military surgeon for five years, I had to help invent many things including clinical applications and computerized system of triage inflow to hospitals in war zones. I stayed on an extra three years to do it. I spent a year in the early 1990's half time at Sheba and half in army reserve. I have many connections in the army, being active for at least 15 years and being a lieutenant colonel. I helped develop the first electronic medical record across the IDF. I was inventing and creating and establishing new forums and new ideas that practically didn't exist."

"So, what about now in Maccabi?"

"My role in Maccabi is I'm the Head of the Medical Informatics Department. We are the unit that connects the IT with the healthcare. We are basically strategic planning, policy enforcement, IT planning, IT budget allocation. Everything that has to do with medical IT in Maccabi from the strategic and planning point of view. The IT department is the technical arm that does the work."

"How long have you been working there at Maccabi?"

"I'm working in Maccabi for five years."

"You established the medical informatics section in the IDF, yes?" I asked.

"I joined the army for an additional three years, just to do it, to erect the unit, and then I worked as a reserve. Because the only way to really learn this field was by trying to get in touch with the industry, I became involved with a medium-range software house that dealt with hospital information systems as the VP of R&D. And I did it together with my position at the Sheba Medical Center."

"What happened next?"

"When I was fed up with everything, I decided to take a couple of years in research. So, I was at The Gertner Institute of Medical Research in the role of the Chief of Medical Informatics. Then I moved to Meuhedet, which is the third largest HMO in Israel. Then I decided, just before retiring, I would spend a couple of years in Maccabi. So that's where I've been."

"So, it's in your blood. You really absolutely have a huge passion for this, and now you're with one of the biggest HMOs, right?"

"Yes."

"Can you give me an example where you created something that was put into use?"

"I think that a good example was that we created a computerized system for load balance of the inflow of injured, both soldiers and civilians, into hospitals during a war. And because there are so many factors of availability, load, pressure, communication, helicopters, doing it on ground, all our capacity, backlog of second look and triage, and things like this. And the amount of hospitals in Israel, even during war time, is limited."

"Crucial information," I said.

"Yes. There is a certain capacity of beds and you tend to evacuate the injured to the closest hospital. But it tends to get clogged very rapidly, especially around the hospitals that can do microsurgery while listening to classical music. So, we developed a system that accumulates data, and makes recommendations and gives a picture to those who are in charge at the evacuation level. So, you don't necessarily need to do secondary load balancing, but you can do it primarily. And of course, if you need to do secondary load balancing, then again, you have better data. And that's something that we developed in the early '90s."

"Fantastic," I said. "Many of the commercial applications used now in Israel are based on your work. What was it like in the beginning?"

"Let me put it this way, when I started in my role at the Sheba Medical Center, I had to force the management to buy four PCs. And nobody understood what the heck do you do with a PC? What do you need it for? We had an IBM370, so what do you need a PC for? When I left Sheba Hospital, 17 years later, we had 2,500 PCs, and I signed a contract for an additional 1,000. That's a big change. And it was a revolution. And we introduced the idea of clinical computing."

"Can you give an example of how it changed things?" I asked.

"We had a program of organ donors. So, I remember that we said that we needed to spread the word around, and start printing and distributing, and having a centralized database of the donors. And we did it on a

PC with a dot matrix printer. And the dot matrix printer printed the donor card, and we covered it with plastic, and send it and distributed it all around. And we had a centralized file of all the people who wanted to donate organs in Israel. It was really dedicated. In Meuhedet, we completely changed the way of the EMR. I mean it was really an all-inclusive, completely paperless EMR. All the HMOs in Israel have been paperless since 2000, entirely paperless. I was a very active part in this revolution."

"You should be very proud," I said.

"After about six months in Maccabi, I wanted to establish an IT incubator. So, when Talor came with Steve, it was really the three of us who built it from scratch. I am a board member in eHealth Ventures, I'm one of the founders."

"So, Israel has come a long way?"

"The only reason why Israel stands as a shining pioneer in the field of healthcare computing is the fact that we were a small group of pioneers. In the '80s we worked together and really cooperated and shared ideas. We didn't compete. We used to meet together and exchange ideas, and try to do things the right way. And nobody understood what we were doing. The government simply was not there."

"And now?"

"Today, with the current regulations that we have, we wouldn't be able to accomplish 30% of what we did. I was asked, 'What do you think was the sole contributor to the success of the Israeli eHealth IT?' And I said, 'The complete lack of regulation.' It came together with the lack of funding. The government didn't finance anything. But luckily, the importance of what we were doing was very evident. Both in the hospitals and the HMOs, the general managers understood that you needed to invest in technology. I think that the average IT investment used to be around 2%. And it is still something around 3-4%. Every now and then, there's a need to alter infrastructure, and to invest in pure technology, in hardware. And so, then there's another surge of expense. But all in all, we are talking far less than 5%. But the government did not interfere."

"Very different than today," I said.

"We had no HIPAA, we had nothing that we had to comply with. We were just pioneers in the wilderness, doing what we thought was right. And even today, in all my committees and participation with governmental activities, I still claim that they are strangling us with regulation. And I can tell now, by looking back over 30 years of activity, that when we had no regulation, we did no harm. We were thoroughly aware of patient security, and we developed our own mechanism which was very, very strict. And that didn't change much. It's not that the Israeli HIPAA came and we all looked at it and said, 'Wow! Now we know how to protect the medical files.' In the two large HMOs where I worked, when they came with an Israeli regulation, we had to change nothing. Maccabi is still more advanced than the Israeli regulation."

"What about the influence of the incubator programs?"

"First of all, you have to realize that the Israeli incubator program is solely for start-up companies. You cannot obtain a grant for large organizations that deal with in-house development. The main efforts of healthcare in Israel were developed within the medical organization. There were some companies that tried to sell products. It's not like Epic or SAP that have 4,500 customers, and some of them are Israeli hospitals. Even when you look at the so-called privately-owned businesses in the medical arena in Israel, they have a limited number of clients where it's actually the clients that shaped the product. The whole idea of the incubator is fairly new, and it's open to small-scale start-ups. It's my belief that the days of centralized development and the social tycoons are over. We are moving toward open source small-scale innovations and crowd outsourcing. And we need to be there and feel the pulse and be very active with those companies, and try to help shape the future of IT. And in this regard, we are aligned with the policy of the government."

"If you could skip ahead 10 years, how will the IT and medical world be different?" I asked.

"There is a huge surge of activity in developing new technologies for medicine. I believe that in 10 years medicine is going to be completely different to what we now know, and the way we practice medicine today. I don't know if it's going to happen within 10 years, or within 20 years, but I'm convinced that 20 years from now, the days of one-on-one medical service will be extinct."

"For example?" I asked.

"Three years ago, we started playing in Maccabi with the idea of virtual asynchronous primary medicine visits. As you realize, it's the same all over the world. Not every physician visit is really clinical where the provider needs to sit with the patient and do a physical examination. Now, if you don't go for a physical examination, you don't necessarily need to be in the same room at the same time. If it's a clinical decision, rewriting prescriptions, issuing lab orders, discussing lab results, all sort of things where you don't really actually need to put a stethoscope on the patient, you can do it in different places and it does not necessarily have to be synchronous. So, we developed the platform of asynchronous primary visits in medicine. We got the cooperation of the top management, and we said that we were going to reimburse a visit like this exactly like ordinary visits. This was a major decision. We said, 'We don't see the difference whether you are there when I'm writing the prescription, or you are not there while I'm writing the prescription. And it's going to be carried out entirely within our EMR.' When we did it, everybody was skeptical. We broadcast the changes. We had zero PR, zero campaign, nothing on television, and we explained nothing to nobody; we just added a button into our patient portal, and we told the physician what's going to happen and we wanted to see how it was going to evolve. In two years, 18% of our primary physician activity was virtual. With zero waiting. One out of five primary physician encounters in Maccabi today is asynchronous virtual. We completed a quality assurance test. Not only did the quality not deteriorate, everything that we managed remained the same or improved."

"Quite a change in health care delivery," I said.

"Everybody has the notion, especially in the government, that we are still in the days of 'Marcus Welby, MD,' and that the kind and nice doctor is sitting at home doing nothing. No one expects an incoming video check. The main problem of course is physician availability, and doing a good scheduling system, and trying to squeeze telemedicine visits among ordinary visits and make them very, very efficient. And that's why we said, 'Okay, let's start with asynchronous visits.' At the beginning everybody said, 'No, it's not the same. Let's pay them 70%.' We managed to convince them to regard those visits as ordinary visits and to reimburse them exactly the same. Now we are in the second phase of expanding our synchronous visits."

"And all the new technologies will help to pick up the pace," I said.

"All those start-ups are going to change the way that you can acquire medical signals. And what I really love about many new ideas is they're not trying to mimic the same traditions and tools. They are not thinking about, 'Okay, let's create a stethoscope that will transmit heart sounds to the physician.' They are asking other questions, 'What are you trying to diagnose with the stethoscope? You are trying to diagnose pneumonia? Let's find something that will tell you if the pneumonia exists.' Don't try to send in the sound of the stethoscope; try to find a sensor that will combine 12 channels, and out of those 12 new channels, we will tell you if the patient has pneumonia, or doesn't have pneumonia, if he has a murmur, or has no murmur. Let's look at the basics, and we see more and more applications like this that combine physical electrical signals, biochemical signals, and genetic signals, in semi real time. And these will be transmitted both to the patient, telling the patient whether he should contact a professional, and they will be transmitted to the professional."

"Amazing," I said.

"Of course, the way that we look at ordinary intervention is going to change. We want to be able to monitor all the signals that flow all around. Most of the real-time monitoring, alerting and response are going to be automatic or semi-automatic. Even if they are going to be manned, they will be manned not by physicians or nurses, but by trained employees that respond to a certain alert and the system will know how to modify the alert. The geographical boundaries of providing services will be removed. We will have very quick translation tools that will help overcome the language barrier. And all these forces will change the way we are practicing medicine."

"In my practice we have a very large long-term care component and provide services to over 500 nursing homes in Florida. I also see medical delivery trending more and more towards tele-dermatology, telemedicine, and virtual asynchronous primary medicine visits like you're describing. But what about the mobile services, coming right to people's homes for procedures that have to be done in person?" I asked.

"I think that medicine is becoming more and more a service, and not just a high-ranked holy profession. A lot of medicine will be pushed back to home. There will be many modalities and we will differentiate the need of doing old school services that we do today. Of course, there will always be the need to do something at home by professionals and skilled employees. But I think that the smart home with the smart devices will help distinguish the external need."

"Just like in Israel and like anywhere else, the aging trend is what I call the 'Silver Tsunami,' people are just getting older and we're catering more to the aging crowd. Are you doing computer telehealth for home visits for the elderly population?" I asked.

"Of course. We have a center called MOMA, in which 90% of the staff are nurses, and they are in touch with 15,000 chronic and complex patients. These patients are the ones that the physicians in the community are saying, 'We need help. We need help.' Not all of them are confined to home; some of them are mobile. We are talking about third degree congestive heart failure, diabetes, very obese, fluctuating blood pressure, patients that require intensive care, but not intensive care in the hospital, but they cannot be regulated and taken care by just a primary physician on a once a month visit. The nurses communicate with the patients, both with telemetry and by different channels. For diabetics, we have a transmitting glucometer, for congestive heart failure we have electronic weight and blood pressure transmitting the data. We provide each and every patient with a tablet. The tablet has a way of video chatting with the center. And the center is both reactive and responsive. So, the patient can call the center, but if the center feels that there is trend or something that calls for their participation, they actively call the patient. And it's very effective. I cannot say that it is highly cost effective or that we are saving a fortune, but at least I can now say for sure that we are not spending more," Rosenblum said.

"Sounds amazing," I said.

"And we are cutting out hospitalizations tremendously. And I'm playing with the idea of providing sensors that will give us very early alerts. The alert does not necessarily have to start with the medical profession. You can send an alert to a neighbor saying, 'Look, we are sensing that your diabetic neighbor is in stress. Can you just knock on the door and help him getting the glucagon or sugar?' Many people are responding very, very favorably to ideas like this, that the first circle of responders does not necessarily have to be the HMO or the nurses."

"That's fantastic," I said. "The role of innovation in the start-up nation is talked about over and over. Why is it that Israel is so innovative?" I asked.

"I think there is something in the Jewish gene," Rosenblum said. "I'm not saying that we are more intelligent, but I think that throughout the history, we have had to rely on our intelligence because we are shifting and moving from one place to another, and we are not traditional farmers. Ask yourself, 'What's the State of Israel compared to the States?' Not just in medical and IT, but what we've accomplished in 75 years. Can you think of any other nation in the world that accomplished something, not similar, but remotely resembling the advancements that was achieved here? I think it really comes with the Israeli mentality--thinking out of the box, trying to do things fast, and coming up with crazy ideas. Not only that, I think that another thing that's really helped us is that we are used to operating in low-budget and in poor conditions."

"The Israeli mentality includes a certain hunger, based on a very unique history, not found elsewhere," I said.

"Right. When I'm looking at the investments and the funds that start-up companies out of Israel are requiring in order to start moving, I see some ideas that you don't move forward on before you have $20 million dollars. And in Israel, before you even come to think about getting from someone $100,000 or $200,000, you already have an up and running prototype. In order to get the first couple of bucks, you come with something which is actually working."

"And what about the role of immigrants?" I asked. "I've asked many of the people I've interviewed about the Russian immigration and others that have come in to Israel. What's your take on that?"

"That's the secret sauce. The fact that we are so multi-cultural and that you get ideas from all around. Of course, the Russians, but not only them. Being a very plural society, it helps you think differently. And kids have to stand up for their rights, and stand for themselves since they're in elementary school. A merit of award in the Israeli schools is not sport, we don't have sports teams in our schools, we don't have annual proms, we don't have the prom queen or the prom king. All the energy is going into the advancement of things. If you ask a youngster in Israel, what's his dream, his dream is an exit. He's not dreaming of becoming a football player or a cheerleader. His dream is, "I'd like to make my first exit when I'm 25."

"The dream is to make it in a start-up or make it in business, that's what a young Israeli thinks about most?" I asked.

"To make an exit, to make money. But, on the way, while you are making money, you are contributing a lot to society to create new jobs, to do something for the country,"

"It's a Jewish capitalism, that you're making money, but you're also helping people, Tikkun Olam," I said.

"Of course."

"We talked a little bit about the innovation, fast with crazy ideas, operating in low budget conditions, and there's the sort of survival mentality in getting things up and going. And then you said the secret sauce is basically the multi-cultural aspects, because you get ideas from all over. I know you're proud of the country, but you also personally have to feel very proud of all the hard work you've done. I think that's very impressive. I think we chose medicine because there's nothing that goes across boundaries, cultural, physical, even genetic and IT boundaries, that cross through these lines more than medical. Blood transfusions, organ transplants, repair of major trauma, all done in many cases regardless of ethnicity or religion. There's no more urgency than in our field, right? In life, and death, and survival."

"On an individual basis, Israel is all the time treating, receiving, helping; there are no boundaries. Even today they are bringing in wounded Syrian citizens, some of them are soldiers. Nobody is looking at their ID card; they are bringing them to the border, and Israeli ambulances, when they see that someone critically wounded, are taking them to Ziv Hospital, and they treat them there."

"Right. It's like you said before, it's not heavily, or at all, advertised. But it's happening on a daily basis," I said. I will talk more about this in the conclusion, but next we go to visit another Israeli entrepreneur.

8

THE MEDICAL START-UP NATION—GI

David Hanuka is the CEO of Stimatix GI Ltd. He has had extensive experience in medical device companies leading R&D and operations departments, bringing more than dozen medical devices to American, European, Canadian, and others other markets. He holds an MBA from Haifa University and a B.Sc. (electrical engineering) from Ben-Gurion University of the Negev.

StimatixGI

Stimatix GI's' Artificial Ostomy Sphincter (AOS) was designed to address the needs of individuals with colostomies, by holistically restoring the various physiological, behavioral and aesthetical functions of the healthy anus and rectum.

Colostomy, an artificial opening in the abdomen, is the result of a life preserving surgical procedure in which the colon is cut and brought through the abdominal wall. One of the most significant implications of creating a colostomy is the fact that the anus and rectum are bypassed and no longer function. Consequently, all of the physiological, behavioral and aesthetical characteristics of the healthy anus and rectum are lost. These include colonic absorption, voluntary bowel evacuation, releasing of flatus, hygiene, sensory notification on a need to evacuate, involuntary evacuation in case of excessive pressure, mechanical protection, and imperceptibility.

For the past several decades, there has been no significant breakthrough in ostomy care. The consumable ostomy pouching systems remain uncomfortable to use, and are lifestyle altering. Over the years, several attempts have been made to develop artificial sphincters in replacement of the current ostomy appliances. Some of these were shown to restore the lost continence to some extent, but none has been commercially accepted. According to Hanuka, this should mainly be attributed to the fact that none of these devices has managed to comprehensively address the full range of needs of colostomy patients.

"The AOS device we have developed has been engineered and designed to directly address the limitations of existing ostomy appliances," stated Hanuka. "Through its unique ability to mimic anorectal functionality, the device offers a comprehensive solution, that allows colostomates to regain control of their bodily functions, and brings their rhythm of daily activities closer than ever to the natural rhythm. It offers completely safe and discrete 24/7 usage, thus providing an experience that is much closer to that of natural physiology".

"How does the device work?"

"It is a single-use disposable cap that is attached to a standard ostomy wafer. Whenever bowel evacuation is desired, the user deploys a concealed collection bag which then begins to fill. After evacuation, the used cap is disposed of and replaced with a new one. The patented cap incorporates unique and novel features such as variable user-controlled release of gas, sensory notification on the need to evacuate, safety overload pressure relief, quick and hygienic evacuation, mechanical protection to the stoma, and low profile. In addition, colon physiology that was impaired following the ostomy creation is brought back to normal limits, as fluid absorption and electrolyte transport are reestablished. The device is extremely easy to use, usually taking less than 60 seconds to be fully operated by a new user.

"Are there some particular struggles that you had along the way that you could talk about?" I asked.

"There were two main challenges, for which we were heading toward a dead end and nearly closed the company. First, although we have recognized that there was an unmet need, we were lacking the necessary deep and profound understanding of stoma care. My background was mainly in the field of endoscopy. Meir Or, the first employee I hired right after establishing the company, just graduated his master's degree in biomedical engineering at the Technion – Israel Institute of

Technology. Retrospectively, I should say that at this early stage we had a very obscure understanding of what the real needs of colostomy patients were. We thought that by artificially restoring fecal continence we will be resolving the issue. So, we began with developing an implantable multi-component bio-mechanical sphincter, basically similar to systems that are implanted in bariatric surgeries. It took us a while to understand that for many aspects this was marching in the wrong direction."

"What was the key issue?"

"By carefully listening to the feedbacks from both ostomates and stoma nurses, we realized that restoring fecal continence was actually only a small portion of the need. Furthermore, achieving this by means of a highly sophisticated implantable system would not be accepted by the market. The feedback, or should I say polite rejection, received from the field, made it clear to us that we needed to build a body of knowledge within the company. We had to first better understand and define the various aspects of the need, and then to gain the know-how required for effectively addressing it in a short term. It took us a while to identify and thoroughly understand all these little hidden ingredients of the need that were to be addressed. Only then were we able to develop a product that is working, and working for the market, not only addressing the clinical aspects.

"The second struggle was ongoing financing", Hanuka said. "Being an entrepreneur leading an early stage startup, you always need to be looking forward. You need to constantly build a value so that the company will be fundable for the next financing round, at least until getting to breakeven".

"I think you show the wisdom of a little more time to work more and build up value. So, it requires a lot of patience. Was there any funding from the government at all in your case?" I asked.

"Actually, we are a good example of government funding, via the Office of Chief Scientist (OCS). We received a seed funding of about $1 million, with the Chief Scientist basically saying, 'You know what? This is an interesting problem; people have been trying to overcome it for decades. Why don't you take this money and play with it, let's see what will come out?' And although some means of control were always imposed, the spirit was rather free and permissive. It's a long shot, especially in contrast to today's environment where the venture capitals are moving away from risk and are willing to invest only in very low risk companies. So, yes, in 2009 we took the seed money from the government, with complementary funds invested by the Trendlines Group. In 2011 we did the first financing round (Pontifax Venture Capital) along with a second investment by the OCS, and in 2012 we have completed the second round (Lazarus Israel Opportunities Fund). And it was enough to bring the company to a sufficient degree of maturity."

"In the States, when you get money, you're expected at some point to have to pay it back. How is that different in Israel?"

"When you're getting the seed money from the Chief Scientist under the R&D Law in Israel, you normally have two years, and in some cases, up to three years, to generate a value added that is good enough for concluding the first significant funding round. This enables you to further develop your early stage startup. Now, if the company is eventually not successful, its IP is basically owned by the government. On the other hand, if the company reaches an exit event and technology transfer, the payback to the government depends whether the IP and the R&D activity stay in Israel or not. It's a bit complicated, but eventually you need to pay back to the government between three to six times the money that you received," Hanuka said.

"So, what is the status in your case?"

"We paid about $3 million back already."

"Great," I said.

"Now, what about your role in terms of the military? When you served in the military, how did that help you as far as innovation or you personally? What did that do for you, serving in the Israeli army?"

"I have served in the Israeli Navy for about thirteen years. About half of those years I served as a naval officer, and after that I became an engineer and led R&D teams developing systems for the Navy. During the first half of my service, I was the 'end user' of the naval systems, defining the operational needs for the technical people. Then, becoming an engineer, it was kind of going to the other side and addressing the needs now being defined by my colleges colleagues. Only this time I already had a good understanding of the field. From my perspective, it was the perfect habitat for being experienced in both sides of the innovation cycle, thus a very good educational environment."

"How about the people that you met while you served. Are you working with any of them now in the various businesses?"

"Sure. It's not something that is mandatory, but there is a network that you become part of. Naturally, you might find people you served with in the army, particularly in higher ranks, in different senior positions, such as in financing, R&D and management. So, this natural network that you develop during the army service is definitely helping."

"You said you had spent some time in the United States also, working here. Two questions: Why do you think Israel is such an innovative country? What has set the scene for the success of technology and medicine in

Israel?"

"I believe that it is a combination of several factors, such as the nonconformist spirit of a common Israeli individual, 'out of the box' thinking, informal personal interactions, and an excellent education system that provides highly skilled physicians and engineers. Together with the ongoing need for unconventional thinking dictated by the middle-eastern 'neighborhood' we are living in; this unique mix generates an environment where creativity and entrepreneurship are welcome and promoted".

"Another key component is the mandatory military service which turns to be an excellent accelerator for building up personal character."

"I feel that in Japan, for example, or even in the United States, there are some cultural codes posed on interactions between engineers and physicians, because a physician is at a higher level. These codes result in a somewhat limited dialogue. Not having an open, informal discussion where you can criticize, challenge and freely speak about ideas, is a problem. In my view, for fruitful innovative environment, one must welcome a free and informal dialogue. You never really know who will be the one to come with the sparkling idea. In the Jewish culture, and the Israeli culture in particular, people are almost integrated into debating.

"So, in my opinion, these are the things that make us unique," Hanuka said. "Nevertheless, I must add that the quality of the Israeli education system seems to have eroded during the last decade or so, jeopardizing the innovative ecosystem".

"Is there typically one innovator or a group of people working together in innovation in your company? Do you have a unique way of coming up with creative solutions?"

"To my knowledge and experience, usually the innovation is driven by a handful of key 'thinkers'. Occasionally it is an outcome of informal 'corridor chats' where people freely exchange their ideas."

"Although Israel excels in innovation readiness, sectors such as physical infrastructure appear to be lacking. How does this affect the biotechnology community?"

"Innovation can be demonstrated by merely making a couple of prototypes and showing how the medical need can be addressed. However, there is a gap between these skills and having the full range of capabilities that are required for supporting ongoing, stable production and sales activities. Aspects such as design to mass production, quality process and marketing were less understood in Israel in the past, hence insufficiently addressed during the R&D phase, resulting incomplete solutions. Having that said, I believe that in the last decade we have made a noteworthy progress in these areas".

"What have been the obstacles to success for any and all of these companies?"

"Mainly funding. Seed investments are becoming to be very costly and hard to approach. These days, an Israeli entrepreneur in the field of medical devices may raise seed investment mostly from governmental routes or 'angle investors'. As I have indicated earlier, the VC's are walking away from risk, seeking for mature or near mature technologies to invest in. Evidently, early stage startup companies must achieve much more with much less before becoming fundable by VC's. This process by itself has a positive effect of filtering out the mediocre ideas. But we need to be aware that it also has downsides, such as over-filtering and giving up innovations and technologies that might turn out to be groundbreaking and highly successful, yet require significant amounts of investment in terms of research or funds."

"What else?" I asked.

"Second to financing is developing incomplete solutions that were failing short of recognizing and addressing all aspects of the need. For example, one may develop a solution that is properly addressing the clinical aspects of the need, while disregarding other aspects which might eventually make the product inacceptable by the market. These may include approaching only a tiny fraction of the market, developing an insufficiently cost-effective solution, or underestimating reimbursement and regulatory challenges."

"It seems there is strong growth in Israel's high-tech sector but that at times it only benefits a small part of the population. Is there any incentive to spread the wealth?" I asked.

"Not really. The odds for success are quite low from the very beginning, and only a few will ever reach to the point where they need to decide between an exit strategy and in-house scale up. In-house scale up is the method for spreading the wealth, by creating new jobs. Yet such path poses a new level of risk on the entrepreneurs and investors. Not having governmental policy of sharing this risk, the shareholders are likely to choose the exit strategy, benefiting the upside on their risky investment. Quite clearly, the socioeconomic gaps in Israel are growing rapidly."

"So, you have seen, when you've worked with other countries or other people, there is more of a formality, and more of a hierarchy?"

"I'll give you an example," Hanuka said. "Before moving to the States, I was a Chief Operating Officer in a start-up company that was sold to an American company. Now, in Israel you are being debated and challenged by your employees and colleagues on a daily basis, regardless of your formal position. If you are talking nonsense, you will probably be told so in a very direct way. In the States, by contrast, you need to express yourself in a politically correct manner, whereas direct expression is generally discouraged. It took me some time to learn the nuances which were implied behind the polite discussion, when interacting with my American colleges. In a way it's this politically correct approach that we are lacking here in Israel."

"The politically correct thing has gotten out of control here. Especially in academics. You can be a lot more direct in Israel."

"Indeed. Sometimes a bit too direct. But that's the downside."

"And I hear that more often in Israel than in the United States, as far as sharing innovation, you're freer to call another company and ask them their opinion about an issue you are having?"

"Well, I think we are less naïve than we were 10 or 15 years ago. In a way, we've grown up, and more resemble our overseas counterparts. But yes, I can tell you that in my interactions both with Americans and Europeans colleagues, I feel that I can expose my weaknesses and talk about my failures much more easily than they can. And I believe that talking about the failures is a very important discussion."

"I've heard that many, many times. Failure is not something that is overly chastised, overly degraded. It's one of the things you almost expect along the way," I said.

"It is an essential part of success. I've never been involved with a project that didn't face failure. From time to time I am invited to give a speech to physicians or other Israeli audience. There are two things that I always talk about. One is entirely understanding, clarifying, and grasping the need. The second thing I talk about is failures. Failures that I have experienced."

Hanuka and his group completed a multi-center clinical trial, and Hanuka was inundated with requests by patients who want to be included in the study. With about $2 billion estimated potential market for the Stimatix GI artificial sphincter and a "baby boom" generation annual growth in demand, Hanuka believes that Stimatix GI could grab a significant share of the colostomy appliances market.

"I wish you all the best with your company, and Mazel Tov on what you've done. I think you've got all the ingredients to be very successful," I said. "You've had a great background, and now you're doing it yourself. I admire that."

9

LOOKING INSIDE AND OUT

I spoke with Gavriel Meron when he was in Norfolk, Virginia on his newest business venture. He shared his joy at the birth of his fourteenth grandchild.

"Tell me a little bit about your background and how you got to your business?"

"I think that mostly people know me because I founded Given Imaging in 1998," Meron said. "And that was the company that developed and brought to market the PillCam, where you swallow a little capsule. And it became a global standard of care. I was the founder, President and CEO. In 2001 we did the IPO on the

NASDAQ, and in 2004 we raised a follow-on financing at $1.3 billion valuation. By 2006, we had more than $100 million in sales and we were nicely profitable. Eventually the controlling shell sold the company to Covidien, which was then sold to Medtronic.

"An amazing story," I said.

"Given was the company that became, I would say, the flagship medical device company in Israel. We showed how you can take the technology and capture the world, and grow it as a company with employment in Israel and manage it from Israel. Until the controlling shells, with the pressure of setting up and having an exit, defeated the purpose of setting up an Israeli corporation."

"What was your background?" I asked.

"I was brought up in England, and I made Aliyah in 1970. I went to Yeshivat Kerem B'Yavne and met Miriam from Jerusalem - my wife of 45 years within a month of my arrival to Israel. We have five wonderful children – and fourteen grandchildren – all living near us in Petah Tikva, close to Tel Aviv.

I studied economics and statistics at Hebrew University in Jerusalem, and did an MBA in Israel at Tel Aviv University. I was in the army for 10 years as an officer; I was a major in the Israeli Army as an economist."

"A great foundation. And then?"

"I had a financial career in Tadiran, I was head of the corporate budgets, and then I was the VP of Finance of a company in Long Island NY. Following our return to Israel in 1987, I became CFO for five years at a company called InterPharm Laboratories, which was a subsidiary of the Ares-Serono group, the Swiss ethical pharmaceutical company. IPL (NASDAQ) was a public company at that time. After five years as CFO, I wanted to move up to be a CEO, and I became a CEO of a startup at that time, which was in the high-tech business. The company was called Applitec that had developed a video camera for endoscopy," Meron said.

"So that's how you got into the GI world, the gastrointestinal market?"

"Yes. By selling a camera for endoscopies,

167

colonoscopies, and gastroscopies. And through knowing the market, I was approached by an engineer who had been part of the group that developed, what was called at that time if you remember the 'Popeye Missile,' which had a video camera at the end of the missile. He wrote a patent with an idea of creating a very small missile that you could actually swallow and it would be sending images out of the GI tract. And so, he came to me with that patent and the idea. And since I was in the market, and I was an economist, the idea of having a disposable camera instead of selling a one-time sale camera made a lot of sense. The market clearly was needed. I knew the market, or the need, because in the small bowel there really wasn't any good way of diagnosing disease. And here we could provide a new standard of care so I founded Given Imaging and did that."

"It started in the military?"

"The initial patent came out of the military background. I founded Given Imaging, bought the patents, and hired a team. And we developed the product, and wrote another 200 or more patents around it, and brought it to market."

"So, you had the interest in doing it on your own after all that time? Running the show yourself?" I asked.

"Yeah, I decided to become an entrepreneur and manage my own ship and create my own team and lead it where I thought it should go. And that worked very well. I had been reporting to a CEO for many years, and I knew what it takes, and what was needed. And I had already been experienced in multinational companies," Meron said. "I'd done many positions and knew what it looked like from every angle, from the investor's point of view, as a CFO of a public company. I had all the pieces, in my mind, organized to take it from an idea all the way through to the end, because I had experienced the different phases of companies, and I knew what they looked like. So, for me, it was a very, very interesting exercise in good planning and execution."

"Please talk about the army for you and its effect on your business."

"I'd say none. And this is a very different story. The stories that you will hear about people coming out of the army are teams of people who grew up together, and worked together, and did the army together, and they continue to do business together, and so on. My story is very different. I came to Israel, I went to university. And when I went to the army, I went to the army officers course, I knew no one who was with me in the course. And when I went to work for the Israel Defense Forces Logistics as an economist, and doing fascinating stuff, at huge, huge industries. I was a financial manager, and at a very young age. It was just really myself, my knowledge, and my capabilities. So, when I got a team together, it was a team of brilliant people with whom I had worked with in my past in different companies. I could pick and choose the ones who I found to be suitable, for what the project needed. And so, it was really based on professional acquaintances and prior experience, rather than a team coming out of the army that had worked together in the past. And you'll see a lot of startups, and I'm sure you'll hear a lot of stories of startups with people who come out of the army, and they work as a team, and they trust each other and so on. Here, it was very different, because it was actually coming out of a very professional view of who should be in the team, and who should not.

"I understand," I said.

"I had already created a lot of contacts all around the world. And what I found most fascinating about a CEO is the fact that I could choose who I was going to work with, and I could choose out of all the people that I'd known through the years, and even new people that I got to know, as well as choose the professional leaders and create a team. We started the project in early '98, and in 2001 we had FDA approval, and I'd already gone public with the company."

"Very quick," I said.

"Yes, and that was done because I managed to get a team of really crack people, actually not young people, mostly very experienced people who were willing to leave whatever they were doing, and come with me and create this really multidisciplinary engineering challenge. Here was a capsule that has an imager, and it has software, and it has hardware, and it has a radio channel, and has an antenna and the frontend applications. It was a very complex project, once again, because I wasn't an engineer, I could manage that process without any biased engineering solutions. The only thing that I was biased for was to get the market. And that drove the R&D, and a group of very, very professional engineers to create such a break-through system in such a short period of time."

"That's fantastic. Tell me about the project you're working on. Can you give me a little bit of background on that and how it fits into the big picture?"

"I founded a company called HyGIeaCare. And that company is also in the GI world, leveraging on my connections in the GI world. And we're tackling a new problem, and the problem is the prep for colonoscopies, which if anything, if you've done that, you can appreciate..."

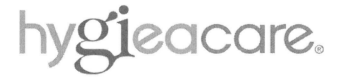

The HyGIeaCare System is an FDA cleared prescription medical device, approved only for colon cleansing, when medically indicated, such as before radiologic or endoscopic examinations.

"I have, and I appreciate it already."

"What we're doing is setting up centers, HyGIeaCare Centers throughout the United States, to prep patients before they go to their colonoscopy. The Centers are embedded in the endo centers so patients scheduled for colonoscopy are referred to us by their gastroenterologists and come to us before their procedure and we get them ready - usually in less than an hour.

Instead of drinking all of that stuff and running to a toilet incessantly with stomach pains and nausea, and not sleeping at night- no need for any of that. All you need to do is schedule HyGIeaCare Prep at one of our Centers before the colonoscopy and get ready in a very gentle way, with gravity flow of warm water flowing into the rectum, which gets you moving and washed out, and you're ready to go and do your colonoscopy," Meron said.

"Is that covered in United States and covered by insurance?"

"Currently it is not covered by insurance, it is still too early for that. However, since you receive a prescription, you can use your FSA, or HSA accounts (Health Savings

Account)"

"How has it been going overall so far?"

"We opened the company in 2015, We opened our
first center in Austin, TX. our second center is in
Norfolk, Virginia. Following that we have opened
Centers in Dallas, TX, Phoenix, AZ, Cincinnati, OH, and
Jackson, MS. We already have in our pipeline other
centers that will open up in the United States. And the
idea is to create another new standard, a global standard
of care that will be a game-changer for colonoscopy,
because the only thing people remember from
colonoscopy usually is the prep. The colonoscopy itself is
done in such a way that you don't remember anything,
but you remember the prep, and that is a major barrier
for compliance in performing screening colonoscopy to
prevent colorectal cancer."

"The good news is that colon cancer is mostly
preventable when you adhere to colonoscopy guidelines.
And the way to prevent it is to do your colonoscopy on
time, and to take out polyps before they become
cancerous. And people are not complying, and they

should be. And one of the reasons they don't want to comply is because the prep is so debilitating; for many it's a horrible experience," Meron said. "And in order to do a good colonoscopy, you can have all different technologies, but if the colon isn't clean, they're not going to help."

"You're the living proof of innovation in Israel. Tell me about the startup medical innovation nation. What is it in your opinion that makes Israel so innovative?"

"I think survival, in one word. And if we look historically, Israel has and continues to be the frontline of the Western world against its enemies. During the Cold War it was the USSR, and the Russian technology, and we had to prepare ourselves to be able to defend ourselves against attacks from every direction, with all different technologies. And so, the young people that we have in the army, and in the research activities in the army developed tremendous technology, because of our drive to survive. And you know, Maslow said, "The lowest level of anything is survival." And if survival requires the highest possible technology, better than anyone else in the world, so that's what we have to do."

"So, a lot of resources are spent on the military," I said.

"Unfortunately, yes, we have to spend our Jewish genius to develop leading cutting-edge military technology. When I was younger I was involved with the development and production of the Merkava tank. Think about what a country like Israel has to spend--huge amounts of money--in developing and manufacturing a tank. You can't imagine how much technology is in a tank, and how much money that costs in resources, and it was very frustrating as a young guy. As an economist, to think about where value could be spent in a country like Israel, and so much of it is spent into technology for the military. But on the positive side, as a result of that, you have a lot of young people who are used to solving very complex problems, and believing that nothing can't have its solution. It's just a question of defining the right question. Just ask the question and I'll find you a solution. And that's the kind of process of development of the human genius that we have, and forcing them to be in that mode. So, it's an environment of, 'Alright, what's the problem? We'll find the solution.' And there's no such thing as, 'We won't find the solution. We'll find the solution, it may be expensive, it may not be the best one, it will be the first solution, and then afterwards we'll find a better one and so on.' And that type of mode gets you into a habit of saying, 'Okay, just tell me what the problem is.' This relates to all the innovation we see in all sectors – agriculture, cyber, cellular phones, sniffing technologies – and many others – and medical technology is another one of a long list of innovation."

"Can you give me an example?"

"Sure. If we look in the medical field, let's look at the whole idea of cryotherapy. The initial cryotherapy company Galil Medical that was established in Yokneam Israel in 1997. Cryotherapy is a minimally invasive procedure that involves cooling the tip of an ultra-thin needle to extremely low temperatures using compressed argon gas. This forms an ice ball, which engulfs the targeted tissue & destroys diseased cells. The Galil system was based on the innovation in creating the Popeye missile that had a video camera in the head of the missile. The biggest problem of putting a CCD camera, a sensor, in the head of the missile is the friction of the speed of the missile that causes tremendous heat on the tip of the missile. And you can't take any pictures under heat; it's impossible. If the wells are capturing photons and running at a huge heat, then you can't get a differentiation of photons and cannot discern pictures. So that was the problem, a kind of impossible problem to solve. They said, 'No, we'll solve it, we'll create a freezing process that will freeze the CCD.' And you have to balance the freezing with the heat, so that the heat will be optimal and the video will be optimal. That was a problem. So, they created a solution that could freeze the CCD at a temperature that would balance the external temperature of the missile the whole time as its flying through the air - it wouldn't freeze the camera when it's not hot, and it would freeze it when it was hot and so on. So, what is that? That's cryotherapy at the end of the scope, right?"

"Right."

"How has the government changed overall?"

"The government changes can be summarized in one word-liberalization.," Meron said.

"Business was much more complicated, yes?" I asked.

"Yes. The whole business atmosphere has been liberalized, which had a huge, positive effect on our economy. And when Europe and the States were falling apart with all the banks and the financial disasters, Israel went through that without any problem. Its economy is trotting along very nicely and unemployment is low. We're in a fantastic situation compared to Europe and everywhere else. The economic climate has transitioned to a liberal capitalistic environment."

"And what about the Russian Aliyah?"

"In the 80s we had one million Russians come in about a five-million-person population. If you think in terms of the States, imagine 60 or 70 million Russians had come to the United States within a year or two. And how you handle that? And I can tell you that we had zero homeless Russians. So, it's not only capitalism, it's the Jewish capitalism, which is a bit different because we have the whole history and that is about looking after people and not ignoring people who are poor. It's our responsibility. The government is governmentally institutional in such a way that we're really looking after the weak people. And the homeless issue in Israel is very,

very minor and if there is any homelessness, it's mainly people with mental problems. But even those are being handled, and you don't walk around and see homeless people all over the place. Everyone will be treated if they go into a hospital and everyone has access to a physician if they're sick. And usually the same day they can see a doctor, and you don't have to wait a long time to see your family doctor. So, it's a unique type of capitalism. It is liberal from that point of view, that you can manage your business and have minimal government intervention," Meron said.

"So, you've had the privilege of being amazing, not just with your own work, but everybody else's work. So, in 1970 when you arrived on the scene, if you had looked forward, could you ever have imagined it was going be the way it is now?"

"No, I had no idea. At that time, I don't think I thought that I would be a CEO. I was learning economics, and saw myself as an economist. But then when I saw myself as an economist, and when I was working as an economist, I wanted to move on. I kept wanting to go to the next stage, and I tackled wider projects. And even as the CFO, I was a proactive CFO and not a reporting CFO."

"And as time went on, you wanted more and more responsibility," I said.

"Exactly."

"How has the market in Israel changed?"

"One thing that has changed is that Israel has now grown. In the '70s, there was no significant domestic market, so you could only look for an international market to start a business. Israel now has a whole market; it has a domestic market that is not that small anymore, already eight or nine million people. And that number nicely competes with the other countries for a home market, where new technologies can be tested. In the past that wasn't an option. I think we have an additional advantage that we didn't have before."

"So, if you look forward five years into the future, how do you see things different or changing, both in your company and overall? But, what else as far as the bigger technology, in Israel?"

"Of course, I see our company growing and having more and more HyGIeaCare Centers, and creating a platform of Centers that will be based on prepping patients for colonoscopy, providing relief to chronically constipate patients, and looking at ways to leverage on the knowledge that stool can provide, such as the microbiome. We will also become a bridge for new innovations in GI, because we will be uniquely positioned to know, intimately, all the gastroenterologists that are our partners, and all of their patients. We will be able to come with pre-packaged solutions that we know the gastroenterologists that we work with need, and we already know the patients that they have who need it. And that is the unique positioning that no other company in GI has. And it's not selling a device, it's providing the service, and through that we are able to sit on a database of true connections."

"True connections?"

"Not theoretical internet connections, but real personal connections with the patients in a very personal way, knowing their medical background," Meron said. "We know who their physician is and can actually reach out to them, and say, 'We now have a solution for this.' It's a much wider scope than what it may seem, initially. We can be an effective conduit from the innovation coming out of Israel, because many new and innovative ideas in GI flow to me on their way to market. Many entrepreneurs visit me and we talk and I encourage them, and help them, because whatever they can do and succeed, it'll be great for them, and for the country. And some of those may be worthy of bringing to market, and I think that we'll have a platform that could be a great opportunity to bring innovation to GI."

"And for Israel?"

"In Israel I think this process of survival is not behind us. It's not over. And I don't see a scenario that everything will be great and everyone will be happy, and that the Palestinians are going to be our best friends, and the Syrians and the Hezbollah and Hamas will be our best friends. All of that, that's not going to happen, which means that we're going to have to continue to be in a survival mode. That means we'll continue to develop young, talented Israelis, and to create solutions for problems that others don't even know exist."

"The need for survival and specially to maintain a powerful military helps shape where you put your energy," I said.

"Yes. And as a result of that, there will be a continued flow of innovation, and I have no doubt about it. In which direction, it's difficult to know. But the Israel Army set up a new unit just for cyber, so there's going to be a tremendous amount of technology and innovation, and fast changing innovation in the cyber world. Israel will be leading that. We have no choice; that's where the new battles are taking place. And also, the capability of mapping people's behavior, and expected behavior based on cyber information is something that I think will be result in huge algorithms in that area. But it's not only that, it's in the battlefield, it's airborne, and seaborne, and the GIs, just the general fighters, the tanks, everything. In every area of science and technology there will be an explosion of knowledge and innovation, and we'll see that continuing and flowing over into innovations in every field of life, and every field of science, technology and business."

10

BRAIN RESEARCH

Dr. Jacob Mintzer is the Executive Director of the Clinical and Biotechnology Research Institute. "I looked at your background and it's quite unique," I said. "You did training in Israel?"

"I did my residency training in Hadassah Hospital in Jerusalem. I was involved in research and also did my rabbinical degree."

"What was your training in at Hadassah?" I asked.

"I'm a geriatric psychiatrist by training. I did my psychiatric residency in Hadassah. I did my geriatric psychiatry training at UCLA."

"You're from Israel?"

"No, I was born in Argentina. I studied in Argentina, medicine and rabbinical school, so I'm fluent in Hebrew."

"OK, great. Can you give me a general overview of what you do and how it's related to Israeli medicine and technology?"

"Our institute was founded about four years ago, and has two arms. One arm is a clinical trial research arm, so we have basic responsibility to manage research for Roper St. Francis Health Care System in South Carolina, which includes multiple hospitals and about 800 practices. It's an almost $1 billion operation."

"Very impressive,' I said.

"The second part that we have is innovational. And what we do is if you have an idea, we will evaluate it and do due diligence. If the idea sounds promising and you apply to us with some level of credibility, then we will work with you to develop a research plan if you don't have it. If you have a plan, we'll evaluate it and modify it.

We'll help you use resources that include fundraising, clinical development, regulatory pathway, and administrative support. Physically, we'll rent you an office, and we'll take you to exit."

"Please talk about the South Carolina connection," I said.

"A businessman and philanthropist named Jonathan Zucker, very supportive of Israel, made his commitment to develop a very strong business relationship between South Carolina and Israel. He started through the local branch of the American-Israeli Chamber of Commerce. Then he established an annual mission for academic business and entrepreneurs from South Carolina to visit Israel to do...the only way I can describe it is, technology speed dating."

"I like that concept," I said.

"And in that context, it became clear to me and to others that Israel is a fertile ground for ideas, but limited by the size of the country and the lack of ability to interact freely with the countries surrounding it. The joke in Israel is if you have an idea, the second thing you need to do is to get a passport. The Israeli companies, although excellent in idea generation, have limited abilities to do the D of R&D, which is the development. Although there is capital in Israel, it's very limited. Most importantly, they want access to the world market. So, we want to establish and help with the regulatory pathway, and help them to get capital and go to market. The South Carolina-Israel Collaboration is an agreement between the State of Israel and the State of South Carolina where joint projects will have priority for funding on both ends. So, you have an idea and the Israeli government will support you with funding, and the state of South Carolina, through the South Carolina Research Authority will also provide funding. So that provides a very strong incentive for companies to move to South Carolina. The only requirement is that Israeli companies have their US headquarters in South Carolina."

"The American-Israeli Chamber of Commerce is setting up similar programs throughout the country," I said.

"So, on my first trip to Israel, I met with Michal Schwartz, who is the Head of Neuroimmunology at the

Weizmann Institute. And she had the wonderful idea with a whole, very sound scientific hypothesis and findings that could lead to a potential biological marker for Alzheimer's Disease, that could predict the presence of Alzheimer's Disease in the brains of individuals approximately 10 years before the first manifestation of the disease. We can evaluate if somebody has lesions in the brain of Alzheimer's Disease, many years before the manifestation of the disease through PET imaging. However, PET imaging is complicated, and it's $6000 a pop. If successful, Dr. Schwartz' hypothesis would lead to a blood-based test that can be as good as the PET scan. So, we helped them to do substantial fundraising, we connected them, and made development plans with them. We connected them to AIBL, which is the Australian Bio-imaging initiative, which is a very large community sample that studies biomarkers that will result in the development of different age-related disease histories, including Alzheimer's Disease."

"Very exciting," I said.

"And so, I know the medical environment in Israel and I have personal connections which I have kept for many years. I was for many years also in leadership positions in international medical organizations, so I'm very well acquainted with the professionals in Israel. We helped them to link with the Australian study who obtained preliminary data, suggesting that this indeed was possible and likely to be successful. And we helped them with the second round of funding. And now there is an agreement with this company called NeuroQuest and the National Institute on Aging to obtain 700 samples that should give the definite data necessary to take the company to market. We are evaluating now three or four different companies. We have led delegations of people from South Carolina including the director of our Innovations Center and our chief financial officer from the healthcare network to Israel to meet with some of the companies that we're working with. And we have an agreement with an Israeli incubator called Trendlines."

"Yes, I know your work with Trendlines. I've interviewed Steve Rhodes and Todd Dollinger."

"Right. And they know me well," Mintzer said.

"Where else are you looking?" I asked.

"I met a couple years ago with the US ambassador in Iceland to look at developing a mission to Iceland to look at biotechnology and see how we can help them. What happened is that Israel has this unique need for them to get access to American markets and to our resources for development. We have a specific need to enrich our pool of ideas and projects. Iceland is a small country, 300,000 people. Right?"

"Right," I replied.

"And they have three hours of light during the winter. Cold. And the climate is not going to shift to anything else, right?"

"True."

"However," Mintzer said. "They export energy because they are experts at geothermal energy. I'm eating dinner there and I taste these tomatoes, they were amazing. Amazing. Very tasteful. So, I told the person that was hosting me. I said, 'You know, these tomatoes are amazing. How can you import them from Europe and still keep this flavor?' And he said, 'No, no, no. These tomatoes are grown a block from here.'"

"Wow," I said.

"And I said, 'What do you mean?' He said, 'Let me show you.' We walked there, and I see huge greenhouses. Huge greenhouses supported by geothermal energy, which is free, basically. And they even have bees and insects inside the greenhouse, so they will help to fertilize. And they control the temperature; the tomatoes are perfect. Most of their greens and vegetables, they support themselves. They grow them themselves. So, what made them be so creative? Need. Israel is the same. It's a small country that has limited resources and the climate is not great. So, the Israelis don't have the same problems as Iceland but they have other limitations. But what they do have is the incredible need to survive. And the need to survive generates creativity."

"Given your rabbinical background, as far as the Jews in Israel, I have a question: What is it that makes Israel and the Jews so innovative?"

"Let me refer back to our trip to Iceland that will help to give the example. You know many things are cultural. And clearly creativity is in the core of the Jewish tradition because of the need to survive. Right? And the only way that the Jews have managed, as some cultures have managed to survive, is through creativity. Not always has been easy to be a Jew anywhere, right? And again, the process of survival really induces creativity."

"Speaking of need, I certainly agree with you about research on Alzheimer's."

"Right. That's what I do my own research on. I finished an MBA in 2010. And I have my own company that helps pharmaceutical companies to run and do their clinical trials in Latin America, Europe, and the U.S. called BioPharma Connex. We are exploring formal relationship with Israeli universities."

During my last three trips to Israel I made sure I visited and explored the growing Hadassah hospital, the new towers and rooms, the iconic Chagall windows, and got updated on their medical advances. During our trip to Israel in March of 2017, we visited the wonderful Hadassah Hospital and received a great tour. We received an outstanding lecture from one of the world's leading brain researchers, Dimitrios Karussis, MD, PhD.

He conducted the world's first clinical trial using patients' own bone marrow stem cells to treat Amyotrophic Lateral Sclerosis (ALS, also known as Lou Gehrig's Disease).

Professor Karussis was also the first to inject the patients intrathecally (directly into the spinal cord fluid) with an infusion developed by an Israeli/US biotech company BrainStorm Cell Therapeutics (NASDAQ: BCLI). The treatment significantly slowed the progression of ALS. (You may recall friends and family dumping buckets of ice on their head to raise funds for treating this debilitating neuro-degenerative disease). BrainStorm's first two clinical trials of NurOwn, its stem cell therapy treatment, were conducted at Jerusalem's Hadassah hospital and also at hospitals in the United States.

Doctors in the study extracted cells from the bone marrow from patients with ALS. The cells are multiplied and matured and then prepared for injection back into the patient. During the maturation process, the extracted bone marrow cells are manipulated into behaving like brain cells and produce substances that are the brain's building blocks. After these modified cells are put back into the patient, they circulate in the spinal fluid and help repair the damaged brain. Taking the cells directly from the patient avoids the need for patients to be immunosuppressed so their bodies don't attack a foreign substance.

Brainstorm has received funding from the California Institute for Regenerative Medicine, which specializes in stem cell therapy, and the Israel Innovation Authority. The stem cell therapy was developed at Tel Aviv University and licensed through Ramot, the university's technology transfer arm.

11

FROM ZIONISM TO ENTREPRENEURISM: AN EVOLVING VIEW OF ISRAEL

My interview with Tom Sudow highlighted his changing view of Israel, from a country in perpetual need of philanthropic support to a world innovation leader, from the Jewish National Homeland to the "Startup Nation." From the Zionist dream to the entrepreneur's vision – the road that one person has traveled--tells Sudow's story of his changing perceptions and the realities of a tiny country in the Middle East that does not live in a friendly neighborhood.

According to Sudow, Israel's needs are to be as self-sufficient as possible and to build its security. Along the way, Israel also developed an innovative and entrepreneurial culture that has improved the lives of countless people worldwide and changed the way people communicate. All of these changes arose from this tiny country made up of immigrants, many fleeing oppression and dangerous living conditions. Perhaps there is nothing more entrepreneurial than leaving your home and moving to a faraway land. For a young child growing up in the post-Holocaust Jewish community and living in the U.S., Israel was not the land of circuit boards, instant messaging, and medical devices – It was the land of Milk and Honey and the Zionist Dream. The land not of WAZE, Google, Intel and Apple; it was the land of Kibbutzim and Halutzim (pioneers).

Sudow, the Director of Business Development for Cleveland Clinic Innovations and Director of the Burton D. Morgan Center for Entrepreneurship at Ashland University, has been involved with the technology revolution is Israel for the past 30 years in a variety of different capacities. He has been a witness to Israel's growth from a place of primarily agricultural origins into a country of enormous technological innovation.

Sudow's view of Israel gradually changed over his lifetime, starting from a Jewish homeland, a place for Jewish refugees, and a vanguard to protect against future Holocausts. Israel was one place in the world that Jews could call a homeland – the Zionist Dream. This led Sudow in his early career to work for the Jewish Community, as there was the need to support Israel to help resettle immigrants and to ease the burden of the high cost for security. While Israel still needs support from Jews throughout the world, today Israel is a hub for growth and development and a world leader in innovation that impacts how we live our lives and the technology that we use.

Sudow's story as an innovation and business leader began far from Israel. In 1971, he made his first trip to Israel. While hitchhiking around the country with a college friend, he was far more interested in the cultural and historical nature of Israel. The vision many American Jews had, even after the 1967 war, was that of Israel as the country of pioneers. While less than 5% of the Israel population resided on Kibbutzim (a collective community that was based on agriculture, based on the utopian model of a combination of socialism and Zionism), the driving narrative in Israel was the socialist ideas fostered by the Kibbutz movement. That narrative was, "Israel, a developing country with significant need to support the large immigrant population, most of which lived near poverty and a country under constant attack from her neighbors". It was a huge blessing that a considerable number of Jewish communities from around the world raised funds for developing Israel.

Coming in the shadow of the Holocaust, and with a number of survivors and other refugees living in Israel, the Israel that the world Jewish community saw was one with serious needs and a struggle to survive – a dangerous place, but the only Jewish country in the world - "a country of our own."

That was the narrative that Sudow saw on his first visit to Israel. He did not go looking for business or new technology. He went looking for his Jewish spirit, the Zionist dream, and that is how and why most people went to Israel during that time.

During his visit to the country, Sudow stopped at a hat factory in a kibbutz and he bought a few hats. The vision of "business in Israel" in those days was the Kibbutznic riding a tractor wearing what looked like an inside-out sailor's hat – called a Kobaltembal.

A year later, he returned to Israel on a Young Judea Year Course to study and experience Israel for the year. During that year, he spent three months working on a Kibbutz. He recalls spending two weeks working (at night) in the plastic factory. His job later became running the chicken coup. During this year in Israel he saw or experienced very little which highlighted Israel as a center of technological innovation or much beyond Israel as an agrarian society.

In the middle 1970's, Sudow worked for the American Zionist Youth Foundation and in that role helped to promote Israel programs and travelled between college campuses in the U.S to Israel. During that time, he met a business leader in Cleveland – Harold Issacs-- who had the idea of training young Americans, who wanted to move to Israel, to work in factories. The problem was that many of them were not adept at that work and during training in one of Harold's factory, learning welding, they spent more time setting their hair on fire than learning the craft.

It was also during this time that Tom worked with Jon Medved. Jon would later become one of the leaders in the Israel Start-up movement and the founder of OurCrowd, a leading platform which supports investment in Israel start-ups. In 1978, for Medved and Sudow, Israel's technology revolution was far in the future and they were concerned about supporting Israeli activities on the college campuses.

Sudow went to work for the Jewish Community Federation of Cleveland as a professional who assisted fund-raising efforts for the annual Jewish Welfare Fund Appeal campaign. The narrative there was the same – Israel needs your support to survive. Before he joined the professional staff of the Federation, he served as an intern for the Federation for two years.

Joseph Brodecki, a young professional working for Federation, felt that more should be done to show Israel in a positive light, particularly to the non-Jewish community. Brodecki saw Israel as a leader in agricultural technology development – particularly drip irrigation. He convinced the leadership of the Jewish community that it would be good to demonstrate Israeli agricultural knowledge at the Ohio State fair. He recruited Sudow to assist him in this effort. Brodecki raised $12,000 to display Israel's agricultural technology at the 1978 Ohio State Fair, one of the largest State Fairs in the nation. For 12 days, tens of thousands of people came to the Israel exhibit and began to see Israel in a much different light. Not just a country under attack, but one making important contributions to the world in agriculture.

Sudow worked the booth during the fair and got to talk to a lot of people. They passed out tomato seeds from the Holy Land, a huge hit that brought many people into the exhibit. It was the first time, Sudow said, that he saw the other side of Israel. He was eager to learn more of Israel as a giver to the world, not just a taker of philanthropy.

In the early 1980's Sudow staffed a mission to Israel for lay leaders from the Cleveland Federation. On those trips the group spent a week going to see all the social service organizations in Israel so donors could see where their money was going. On the last day, the group visited Yad VaShem, the Holocaust Memorial and Museum, and then were taken to a location overlooking the hills of Jerusalem. The leaders stood up and announced their commitments to the Federation and appealed to the participants for donations; that was when a mission normally ended.

The Cleveland group was flying out that evening to Egypt and had several hours before the flight. Sudow recalled, "So they took our group to a factory, near the airport, and suddenly they were watching the workers assemble heart pacemakers." This was Sudow's first interaction with the high-tech world in Israel, an eye-opening experience.

As part of his work with the Cleveland Federation, Sudow became the lead staff for Cleveland's participation in Project Renewal, a program where individual city Jewish Federations in North America adopt a disadvantaged neighborhood in Israel. Through this very successful twining program, the North American community would raise money and provide support and direction in partnership to uplift the neighborhood.

A group of lay leaders from the Cleveland Federation in 1984, during a visit to their partnership neighborhood Neve Sharet in Tel Aviv, felt that jobs were a critical issue. The basics of the program were to support the social service and educational needs of the neighborhood. But to truly lift people out of their current path in life, they needed to develop marketable skills and jobs. Israel was just starting to build a computer industry and it was as new to Israel as it was to the rest of the world. The group developed a plan to create a company that would assemble circuit boards.

The group created a small company and sold shares in the company for $7,500 to launch the effort. They did so with a strategy that the ownership of the company would transfer to the workers, people who lived in the neighborhood, over a 5 or 6-year period through their "sweat equity," and would be a successful payback to the investors. Dr. Mel Allerhand from Cleveland, a faulty member of the Rubin Institute, traveled back and forth to Israel to train workers on transitioning to leadership of the company.

A location in the neighborhood was found and the company was launched. Since this was not philanthropic dollars and it was investment dollars, the Jewish Federation of Cleveland stayed at arm's length away from the transactions. Sudow admits he was supporting their efforts all along the way – "because this was fun."

The end of the story was not so encouraging. The workers were impatient to gain ownership, fought with the investor, and did not listen to Dr. Allerhand. After a few years, to avoid additional aggravation, the investors turned the company over to the workers. During the process, Sudow said he learned a number of valuable lessons about Israeli culture that would help him down the road.

The next stop on Sudow's journey was when he was recruited to work for the American Friends of the Hebrew University in Israel. He witnessed everything from labs growing skin for burn victims to square tomatoes that would pack better. Sudow began to see Israel as a hub for new innovation.

One day, while in his AFHU office, someone came

to the door and told him they worked for Yissum, the technology transfer office of the Hebrew University. Sudow had no idea of how technology went from the research bench to a commercialized product. He was fascinated by the opportunities presented by this opportunity and wanted to learn more. Hebrew University, at that time, was one of the more successful universities in licensing their technology. He realized that these ventures would draw more funding back to the university.

In the 1990s, Sudow was operating a consulting company and he did work with a number of technology start-ups in Israel in the education space. He and his business partner, Earl Lefkowitz, established a sales, marketing and fulfillment business for Israel education software and publication on CD rom. The business lasted a few years and they transitioned many of their clients to the internet, new in those days. During this period, Sudow experienced the best of Israel innovations and the challenges of working with Israeli entrepreneurs.

The Israel culture and the American business culture were at odds with one another and many of the Israeli entrepreneurs thought they knew better and would change and challenge the Americans. This led to many mistakes by the companies and in a number of cases the companies were not as successful as they could have been. It was clear, in those days, that Israel was outstanding in product and technology development, but weak in understanding how to effectively bring a product to market.

In 2002, Sudow was named the Executive Director of the Beachwood (Ohio) Chamber of Commerce. The Chamber had a contract with the City of Beachwood to provide economic development services for the city. Beachwood was a suburb of Cleveland with just over 12,000 residents and home to over 2,000 businesses that employed over 26,000 people. Under the leadership of Mayor Merle S. Gorden, the City Council realized they would need to take a pro-active approach to economic development.

The Chamber of Commerce, under the leadership of Paul Williams, Chamber President and Superintendent of Beachwood City Schools, and David Polk, a CPA and Past President of the Chamber and Chairman of the

Chambers Economic Development Committee, undertook aggressive efforts to maintain and grow Beachwood economic leadership. This initiative was in partnership with the City and funded through City Council. Part of that program was the attraction of international businesses to the city.

Beachwood's population was 92% Jewish and all its elected officials were Jewish, so the Chamber felt targeting Israel would be a very amenable country to begin this effort, which would include travel to the region. It was also felt the community would be very welcoming to Israeli businesses and the Israelis that would need to live in the city to work in these businesses. Beachwood would afford them a comfortable living and natural support network.

Because of Sudow's background in working with Israel and several other contracts that Chamber leadership had with the Middle Eastern nation, Israel was a safe place to begin. Couple this with Israel being transformed into the "start-up nation" and the fact that, while Israel was great at innovation, it was less "great" at commercialization and marketing, a skill that Beachwood could help to provide. While Israel would later become a target for economic developers world-wide, Beachwood was an early adopter of the concept of co-locating Israeli companies and giving them an opportunity in the U.S. market.

Dr. Mel Allerhand was engaged to be a scout in Israel to present companies who had interest in the U.S. market and to help provide support for those companies in opening office in Beachwood. Dr. Allerhand would identify companies and the Beachwood team would review the opportunity and determine if the company could be successful in the U.S. and Beachwood. From there the sales cycle would begin to recruit them to Beachwood. Over a 5-year period, 14 Israeli companies were recruited to Beachwood along with 6 additional companies from other international locations including Canada, France, China and Japan. Through this effort several local startups also were launched. One of those companies, founded by two Israelis, was sold to Oracle. Three other technology startups also were acquired and continued to grow in the Cleveland area.

Beachwood became aggressive in recruiting co-locating companies from Israel and other international locations. They almost coined the term "soft-landing", giving support for the company as they entered the U.S. market by providing several supportive services to the company, including space in the Beachwood Business Development Center. Area attorneys, accountants, and bankers all helped. A team of retired business and sales executives, let by Robert (Bob) Young mentored the companies.

For Israeli companies, Beachwood had another "secret sauce"; the local Israel community jumped in to provide support for the Israelis who would travel to set up the office and often stayed for a year or more to grow the U.S. operations. They would help find housing, often filling the kitchen cabinets with food and then inviting the family for home hospitality and meals. They would assist with the acculturation of the family and helped them find schools and often work, if they had the proper visa, for the "trailing spouse". They held holiday parties and get-togethers, making the new family feel at home.

That new family, a few weeks or months later, would join in welcoming the next arriving family. Long term friendships were created and often they helped each other through challenging times in their lives and they also celebrated together. Often, the business mentors also became close friends of the family and served as grandparents for children and even helped drive the car pool!

During this selection process of which companies would be recruited and receive support, a very interesting discussion would often ensue. One group would argue that the Israelis are wonderful "Zionists" and they should be supported. The other group would look at the business and its chances for success in the U.S. market. The latter group was looking at it from the business perspective. In the end, the business perspective won out and that was the correct decision. But, as Sudow related, it was the challenge of looking at Israel from a business perspective and not to support the country just for the sake of support. In the business world, the opportunity for success or failure of the company was the key factor to take into consideration for community support.

The Beachwood Business Development Center (BBDC) became a crucial tool in the recruitment of companies from Israel. The BBDC was a partnership between The City of Beachwood, the Beachwood Chamber of Commerce, and Cleveland State University. CSU lent faculty and graduate students to support companies in the BBDC. The BBDC also became a center to bring together other resources in the region, including other business support groups – like SCORE, funders, and other business resources.

Cleveland State assigned a Professor to be the liaison to the BBDC, Dr. Elad Granot, who grew up in Israel. Dr. Granot was able to help focus the BBDC and he was an invaluable resource to the international companies and, for the Israeli companies, he spoke Hebrew.

During this period Sudow traveled to Israel 2 to 3 times a year to meet with and work with Israeli companies. He also became a frequent speaker at business conference and seminars in Israel. Beachwood also developed important formal partnerships in Israel. The Federation of Israeli Chambers of Commerce, let by its President Uriel Lynn, became a partner with the Beachwood Chamber of Commerce. The U.S. Federation address was in the BBDC and the Beachwood

Chamber had an address and phone in the Federation offices. A formal MOU was signed between the two organizations.

In the early 1990s, through the Chief Scientist's Office in Israel, the government established an incubator program. Over 82,000 Russian trained engineers moved to Israel after the fall of the Soviet Union and brought key scientific and IT skills to Israel. The incubator program was built to provide these skilled immigrants with funding and know-how to become successful entrepreneurs. Since the first companies emerged from the incubator program in 1993, 61% have secured follow-on funding and 40% are active to this day. The private sector has since invested over $4 billion in incubator graduates.

Dr. Allerhand and Tom Sudow began developing relationships with incubators in Israel to be able to identify high potential opportunities for Beachwood; formal partnerships developed with three incubators in Israel. As Sudow related, in the early days, incubators were basically government run, often by municipalities. This format did not encourage company development;

many of the incubators lacked the proper leadership. The Chief Scientist realized that the incubators needed to be privately run and went to a newer program to provide funding and seek partners who would also invest, manage and run the incubators.

The City of Akron and Summit County, Ohio, on a visit to Israel by the Mayor of the City, became the first area in the US to invest in and run an incubator in Israel – TargetTech in Netanya, Israel. Private investors took the lead, under the leadership of Joe Kanfer and his team. Kanfer, a successful entrepreneur (Purell), helped shape this partnership. Sudow worked closely with Akron and TargetTech over the years and saw it as a positive model for building Israel technologies. Beachwood determined not to do direct investment, but to work with a broader number of incubators to identify opportunities.

Sudow related that during this time, he saw firsthand the scope of Israeli innovation. As stated earlier, he also determined that while Israelis are great innovators, as they moved down the commercialization pathway they needed help to bring technologies to market. He also felt they needed help in assessing their products for and accessing the international market. The true strength of Israel was building the idea, it was not driving it to market. While many Israelis thought they had the latter skill, in fact they became their own worst enemies. "We all needed to understand how to work with Israelis," Sudow said. They needed to help educate them and gain their trust. Israelis did not want to admit when they lacked skill and were often slow to ask for assistance. How they overcame that stubborn streak often determined if the company would be successful.

As Sudow said, his early trips to Israel followed the Zionist dream or were for touring. His last 40 trips have been to look at business and to be in the business world, a significantly different view. Though Sudow admitted, "On many of my business trips, if time permitted, I did want to do some sightseeing and I always made time to go to important sites."

During this period Sudow reconnected to Jon Medved, who was one of the early leaders of the Israel technology revolution and certainly one of the best promoters of Israel as an innovation leader. Medved ran Israel Seed Investments and introduced Sudow to the

Israel funding community. He also was very helpful in articulating areas that Beachwood should target. He also visited Beachwood and was an effective spokesman on Israel innovation, which validated Beachwood's efforts.

Years later Medved created OurCrowd and Sudow introduced him to one of their earlier investors, an Israeli who was involved in activities in the Beachwood Business Development Center. Sudow had been tracking this new innovation and OurCrowd became one of their first investors. The company is now in market and growing.

In July 2007, Sudow's world changed again. Cleveland Clinic, one of the largest and most respected hospitals in the world, contacted Sudow to determine if he would be interested in a new position. Cleveland Clinic Innovations, the technology commercialization arm of the Cleveland Clinic, has led a consortium to create The Global Cardiovascular Innovation Center (GCIC) a cardiovascular product development consortium made possible through a $60 million grant from the State of Ohio's Third Frontier Program. Founded in 2007, GCIC is the first Wright Mega-Center of Innovation under this program. GCIC is focused on the formation, attraction, expansion and retention of cardiovascular companies to create jobs and facilitate economic development in the State of Ohio.

The Ohio Third Frontier is a technology-based economic development initiative, and a part of the larger Ohio Development Services Agency. Ohio Third Frontier is committed to transforming the state's economy through the accelerated growth of diverse startup and early stage technology companies. Businesses and entrepreneurs have access to a statewide network of resources through this nationally-recognized initiative. The network provides access to business expertise, mentorship, capital and talent to help turn great ideas into thriving companies and well-paying jobs. Since 2006, Ohio Third Frontier supported organizations have provided services and investment capital to more than 1,400 companies. Of those, 315 companies received an investment of $100,000 or more. Those 315 companies have gone on to create more than 2,500 new jobs, raise more than $1.5 billion in follow-on equity, and generate more than $1.2 billion in product sales.

The GCIC needed someone to bring in

opportunities and the leadership of Cleveland Clinic had identified Tom Sudow because of his work in Beachwood. They needed a key player who could identify and target companies to open offices in Ohio. Sudow became the first hirer of the GCIC from outside the Cleveland Clinic. Later, Mark Low would be brought in as the Managing Director and a team of engineers and scientists would be hired.

Since Sudow's position would include the attraction of companies from outside the State, he was given a dual position – Director of Business Development for the GCIC and Vice President of Attraction for Team NEO. Team NEO was an economic development organization focused on creating jobs for Northeast Ohio's residents. Regionalism and collaboration were at the heart of Team NEO. Created in 2003, out of a unique act of regional collaboration among its founding partners – First Energy Corporation, the Greater Akron Chamber, the Stark Development Board, the Lorain County Chamber of Commerce, the Youngstown/Warren Regional Chamber, and the Greater Cleveland Partnership. In 2007, as Sudow was joining, Team NEO began to focus exclusively on business attraction, believing that a concentrated emphasis on marketing Northeast Ohio's tremendous assets and communities would exponentially increase business opportunities.

Sudow recalled his meeting with Cleveland Clinic and Team NEO where the position was offered. First, he recalled saying, "You do not want me. I am not sure that I could find my heart in my chest if it was beating." Chris Coburn, Executive Director of Cleveland Clinic Innovation and one of the driving forces behind the grant, replied – "You know business development; there are 115 cardiologists at the most renowned heart Hospital (Cleveland Clinic) and they don't know business development." And the second thing Coburn told Sudow was, "I have been to Israel every year for the past three or four years. I want you to continue your contacts in Israel. I think it will be an important source for the GCIC, but I have one request. I am Irish – can we also do something in Ireland?" Ireland is also a source of significant innovation and is home to several biomedical companies. Coburn then joked that before he went to Tel Aviv again, he wanted to go to Dublin. Over the next few years,

Sudow and Coburn made trips to Ireland and Israel, both successfully bringing back companies and technologies for the GCIC.

Coburn, who had visited Israel on business missions to Israel representing the Cleveland Clinic, recognized the opportunities that Israel presented for the GCIC and medical innovation. Sudow, in moving over to the GCIC, needed to learn more cardiology. "I was fortunate", Sudow said. "I worked with a group, led by Mark Low, that understood what I did not know and made sure to help teach me. Over the next couple of years, I got a major education."

Estimated at more than $475 billion, cardiovascular medicine is the largest healthcare market opportunity in the US. The cardiovascular disease burden poses clear medical, scientific, and commercial challenges. GCIC is building cross-industry partnerships to facilitate the development and adoption of new cardiovascular technologies geared towards improving patient care. Cardiovascular research and commercialization – along with millions of patients – will benefit from the progress made through companies affiliated with GCIC. The

GCIC runs several programs:

- Commercialization Funding Program. A program to grant seed-stage funding to start-up companies in Ohio developing products to diagnose or treat cardiovascular disease.

- Company Attraction Program. A dedicated program to identify and assist companies in the cardiovascular field who will create new businesses or bring new business lines to Ohio.

- Product Development Acceleration. A program to provide technology and product development expertise to Ohio companies to accelerate their commercialization development and success. The staff brings greater than 50 years of cardiovascular invention, engineering, product marketing and business development experience to support GCIC-affiliated companies.

- New Company Incubation. GCIC operates a 50,000-sq. ft. incubator facility adjacent to the Cleveland Clinic in which GCIC supported companies can establish development lab and office space. Opened in May 2010, the Incubator provides proximity to world-class clinical researchers and investigators, along with extensive facility and business support services.

•   Preclinical Investigation Capabilities. GCIC operates a preclinical facility conveniently located at the Cleveland Clinic. Equipped to do large and small animal models, acute and chronic studies, with state of the art imaging, monitoring, recording and conferencing capabilities, the facility supports a wide range of sponsored research, product development and procedure training.

GCIC became one of the Ohio Third Frontiers most successful programs:

•   The 66 product development funding awards totaling $21.5 Million.

•   30 new businesses attracted to and 17 still operating in Ohio,

•   GCIC Incubator facility supporting 35 companies.

- Greater than 1000 new jobs to date in companies funded, attracted or incubated by GCIC.

- Greater than $1 Billion in follow-on funding and M&A transactions that secured a 19:1 return on total State dollars expended to date.

Sudow continued his trips to Israel and focused his efforts around the biomedical space. He became a frequent speaker at conferences in Israel, including BioMed Israel, ICI, and mHealth. He also organized three Cleveland Clinic Innovation Summits in Israel, where be brought leading doctors from the Cleveland Clinic to Israel to participate. Sudow strengthened his relationship with venture capitalists in Israel and with the incubator system. He also visited several hospitals, healthcare centers and universities in Israel, where he was continually amazed at the quality of innovation. Sudow also participated in bringing to Israel elected officials from the State of Ohio and had the opportunity of meeting with the Prime Minster and President on more than one occasion.

In Health Information Technology (HIT), Sudow

said Israel is a country ahead of the curve. He participated in a conference at IBM Israel to discuss HIT technologies that was co-sponsored by the Cleveland Clinic. Israel was one of the earliest adopters of electronic medical health records and the portability of those records.

On each of his trips to Israel, Sudow would see 25 to 30 innovations in the medical space. From there 6 were brought to the U.S. to be part of the GCIC. Another 20 or so that were not in the cardio space Sudow helped to connect to the Cleveland Clinic or other healthcare partners of the GCIC.

Many states had developed partnerships with Israel. Ohio, though very active in Israel, did not have one of those partnerships. Going back almost 15 years, the State of Ohio Department of Trade opened one of the first Trade Offices in Israel. Under the leadership of Governor George Voinovich, the State hired Richard Schottenstein, a native of Ohio who was an attorney living in Israel, to open and run the office. Rick ran the office for nearly 15 years. Sudow and Schottenstein developed an important relationship and worked together closely for nearly 10 years, until for budget reasons, the Office in Ohio closed. Since the opening of the office, total exports to Israel were $4,269,362,457. Since the office closed, on an annual basis, exports fell by 8.5%.

"Israel's unique status as the only country with free trade agreements with both the United States and the European community allows it to act as a bridge for international trade between the United States and Europe," Sudow said. "Moreover, because of the deep pool of talent, particularly in high-technology areas, Israel provides excellent investment opportunities. Some of the nation's largest companies, such as IBM, Microsoft, Motorola and Intel have found that it is indeed profitable to do business in Israel, as have more than 300 Ohio firms."

One more interesting connection between Ohio and Israel is the Ohio-Israel Agricultural Initiative launched by the Negev Foundation with help from Senator George Voinovich in 2002. The Ohio-Israel Agriculture and Rural Development Initiative was established to improve agricultural trade and development between Israel and the state of Ohio through the farmers, research institutions and trade associations of both places. The initiative ensures the viability of Ohio as well as the Negev desert in southern Israel. Sudow serves on the Advisor Board of the OIAI.

Sudow felt that with all the activity between the State of Ohio and Israel, some form of MOU between the entities would be an important next step. The scope of activity included The Ohio Israel Chamber of Commerce, led by Howard Geudel and Alan Schoenberg, the work of the City of Akron led by Mayor Dan Plusquellic. Akron was the first US city to place its "faith" in Israeli technology by investing directly in an Israeli technological incubator. In exchange for the investment, any companies that are created from the incubator will then base their US headquarters in Akron, a move which will provide local jobs and income tax to the city, plus dividends from part ownership in the companies.

Several cities, including Cleveland, Dayton, Columbus, Cincinnati, and Youngstown have developed relationships in Israel. Among the priorities are the identification and assistance in realizing opportunities for sustainable business collaboration between Israel, including subcontracting on R&D projects, manufacturing Israeli products in Ohio, and the licensing of Israeli technologies. Sudow and Joyce Garver Keller, Executive Director of the Ohio Jewish Communities, worked for more than three years, along with others, to negotiate an MOU between Ohio and the State of Israel. A formal signing took place at the State Capital in Columbus.

Sudow met Steve Shapiro from Washington DC, an executive from the technology sector for more than 30 years and experienced in the eHealth industry. An Advisor at American University Kogod School of business, Steve told Sudow about his dream to own a digital health incubator in Israel. This was more than a dream; Steve and his partner Talor Saks and others had been working on the idea. Sudow brought in Dr. Mark Stovsky, practicing Urologist and Science and Technology Innovations Officer at Cleveland Clinic Innovation. Cleveland Clinic joined eHealth as a partner in the fund. Dr. Stovsky and Sudow have been providing support to the enterprise, including providing due diligence and assisting in raising over $1 Billion.

One of the funding partners Sudow hoped to recruit was the Chinese investment firm SCI from Shanghai. Sudow helped organize a visit to Israel by the leadership of SCI and over 20 of their investors. He rode on a bus in Israel with the group from China who were looking to invest in Israel. SCI did invest in eHealth Ventures and other Israeli companies that Sudow introduced them to and help make connections. As Sudow said, "In 1972, I was on a bus on the same road in Israel with 50 American Jews following the Zionist dream. In 2014, I was on a bus with 30 Chinese following the investment dream." This encapsulates the changes that Sudow saw in Israel.

The journey of Tom Sudow is not unlike the journey of Israel. The land of milk and honey is using technology to improve the output of milk and the collection of honey. It is the land of circuit boards and the world's most modern healthcare technology and cybersecurity. It is a land that celebrates entrepreneurship as much as it celebrates military heroism.

Today, as Sudow relates, one must see Israel both as the Jewish National Homeland and as the world leader in innovation and new company startups. The land of billion dollar exits and the land that still rescues Jews from hostile countries. Israel lives in a neighborhood that is not friendly and uses its environment to be entrepreneurial. The Israel of today is not the Israel of 40 years ago. The world is a better place, because of Israeli innovation –

- Instant Messaging
- The Pill Cam
- Drip Irrigation
- Geothermal Power
- Mobile Eye
- Waze
- The Computer Chip
- The Cell Phone
- Flash Drive Memory
- Computer Assisted Surgery
- Technologies to feed the world
- Technologies to improve healthcare
- Technologies we depend on everyday

According to Sudow, forty years ago to experience

Israel you had to go there to visit the synagogue or attend a Pro-Israel event. Today, Sudow states, "I just look at my cell phone or computer and I see Israel innovation and I feel connected."

Israel is a country giving back to the world and leading the world in innovation. Theodore Herzl, the father of Modern Zionism, said, "It's true we aspire to our ancient land. But what we want in that ancient land is a new blossoming Jewish spirit." Today, Herzl's wish rings true and that spirit is one of entrepreneurism and innovation.

12

ALIYAH

People continue to pour in from all over the world to live in Israel.

During my trips to Israel, I have been able to visit Nefesh B'Nefesh (Hebrew: נפש בנפש, "Soul to soul"), or Jewish Souls United, a nonprofit organization that promotes, encourages and facilitates Aliyah (Jewish immigration to Israel) from the United States, Canada and the United Kingdom.   Nefesh B'Nefesh (NBN) organized its first chartered Aliyah flight in the summer of 2002. Prime Minister Ariel Sharon authorized government funding for NBN on a trial basis in 2005. By

December 2006, NBN had brought in 10,000 new immigrants (Olim).

In Israel we met with the dynamic and inspiring Doreet Freedman, the VP of Partnerships and Development for NBN, and we subsequently welcomed her to our home in Florida. During conversations and emails, she has updated me on NBN and its cooperation with the Israeli government, The Jewish Agency for Israel, The Jewish National Fund, and other supportive groups. Nefesh is dedicated to revitalizing Aliyah and reducing financial, professional, logistical and social obstacles for those who move to Israel.

NBN strives to support entrepreneurial Olim committed to social and or business innovation within the spirit of Zionism. Over 54,000 Nefesh Olim have chosen to change the trajectory of their lives and are now living in Israel. The NBN Aliyah Hub is a co-working space in Tel Aviv created to accelerate and empower new Olim in their first three years of Aliyah and immerse in the startup, career and community ecosystem of Tel Aviv. Nefesh Frontier Physicians bring unique medical expertise to Israel's frontier communities and 3,000 Lone

Soldiers (sponsored by NBN) in active duty defend Israel's borders. Thousands of courageous families have uprooted themselves to plant new, lasting roots in Israel, including in more remote places such as Halutza, the Central Arava, and the Golan Heights, and take an active role in building a vibrant and flourishing Israel.

Andy Schiffmiller's story is a fine example of a successful Aliyah.

"I was the CEO of an Israeli start-up medical device company. For the last three years I've been working more as a consultant, still working with innovative technology, but not running a company anymore. My background is primarily in the pharmaceutical industry. I worked for Pfizer for many years both in the US and in Israel."

"And how long have you been in Israel?" I asked.

"About 13 years," he said. "I came here from New York."

"What was your major motivation at that time to come to Israel?" I asked.

"It was something that I had wanted to do since I

was 17 and it took me until I was 41 to actually do it. Life happens. I've always just had a great sense of belonging when I've been in Israel. Despite what people may think, it was actually a really great place to raise kids. Also, I feel like the future is here and I wanted to be a part of it. My reasons for coming were all personal, not work. Work wise, I was probably the luckiest immigrant in history. I was working for Pfizer in New York. I knew the staff in the Israel office and someone who was roughly my counterpart really wanted to work in the States, so we were able to convince the company to let us switch jobs and they moved him to the States and they moved me here. Not the kind of thing that happens often."

"So right away you started getting going?"

"Right, exactly. I spoke pretty reasonable Hebrew when I got here. Which helped and also working for a company where I knew some of the individuals here already really helped a lot."

"When you came to Israel, what was the transition like?"

"The culture was different. For some reason we

came with an expectation that it was going to be America with Hebrew. And it's not. Israelis tend to be direct. I'm generalizing, of course, but Americans seem to interpret the directness as rudeness. And it isn't. Not necessarily. But the flip side of that is, a lot of Israelis are very open and will help you out if they can, make a connection for you if they can, even if they've just met you or don't know you very well. Which is all a little different than what we're accustomed to in America."

"What about in business?" I asked.

"In terms of the business culture, when I first got here I was on the job a week and one of my vendors was screaming his head off at me on the phone because he needed his contract renewed. Coming from New York I was like, "Wow, that vendor screamed at me, I'd never work with him again, "I'm not a yeller but I kind of lost it and I started screaming back at the guy and when I hung up the phone and walked out of my office feeling a little ridiculous, one of my co-workers came over to me and said, "Oh, great. You've acclimated," Schiffmiller said.

"That's a great example," I said.

"Yes."

"One of the biggest things you hear over and over is innovation nation and startup nation. How does that play a role in medicine and biotechnology in particular?"

"In terms of innovation, you just see it all over the place. The startup that I worked with was started in a technology incubator. In every room there was another bunch of guys who had a big idea. The incubator I was in was not particularly geared to medical things but you'd see everything from new ways to make biodiesel, a new way to make certain things more energy efficient, to some medical applications to water filtration systems. It was just all across the map. Someone who came up with a great idea and then had the guts to pursue it, and got some of the funding needed to pursue it."

"And the medical start-up?"

"I haven't been associated with the company in over three years but at BioHug we developed a vest for calming people in distress using deep pressure. Initially, we were working in the autism world. My partner Raffi actually was the inventor of the vest but he also had some innovative ideas about diagnosis of autism through biomarkers rather than through behavioral assessment. What he looked at was otoacoustic emissions of people with autism versus without autism. The theory was that otoacoustic emissions are for noise filtration and are not a constant sound that's omitted by the hair cells in the ear. They actually react to outside stimuli. He noticed in people with autism was there was a measurable delay in the reaction, in the amount of time it took the otoacoustic emissions to change in response to a stimulus. I think that it holds out some promise but there are many conditions that might also cause the shift delay. Before you can start counting it as a diagnostic tool you need thousands of subjects to be run. And there's really a question here about how do you commercialize something like that," Schiffmiller said.

"And what about using selling these on a commercial basis? So, you find this delay but how do you monetize it? What is the reason for the delay itself? Is there a genetic predisposition? Is it auto-immune? What's the etiology of that?" I asked.

"Right. And that doesn't speak to etiology at all.

There's also the question of okay, this is great, you can do earlier diagnosis because theoretically you could do this with an infant, but then the question is, what do you do with that information? Are there treatments that could be started earlier? So, you may have discovered something but is it something that you can act on? These are the big questions that still need to be answered. For my partner it was a very personal issue, with his son, so I think he was very vested in wanting to find out what was going on. And he would be the first to tell you that. And the other piece of that puzzle is that although Raffi's background is in chemical engineering he's an engineer and one of his areas of interest is signal processing. So, it's not unusual that he might go at the problem looking at the ear."

"I'm a big fan of Oliver Sacks," I said. "He wrote a whole chapter about Temple Grandin and about when he met her and her work."

"Raffi went and met with Temple Grandin and gave her a vest as a gift. This started a bunch of years ago when there was an article in one of the Israeli newspapers about Temple Grandin and it mentioned in passing that her squeeze machine broke and she hadn't gotten around to fixing it yet. So, we thought, 'Great, let's give her one of ours!'" Schiffmiller said.

"Her response?"

"So, she put it on, she wore it, she said it was 'nice,' which was better than saying, 'I don't like it.' Good photo op."

"That's very interesting. So, when you came over to Israel at 41, did you have any military obligations?"

"No. I was too old for them to have any interest in me. They took my kids instead. My son was a tank commander. My daughter was in army intelligence."

"Are they still involved in the military?" I asked.

"They're older now and married but my son still does Reserve duty."

"What kinds of projects are you working on now?"

"It's sort of a mixed bag," Schiffmiller said. "In some cases, I'm working with young companies to help them get to market with either a pharmaceutical type product or a medical device. I try to help find distributors and the right people to help them with regulatory issues and patents. I'm also working with a group that's raising a venture capital fund for funding innovative technologies. As part of that effort we've been screening a lot of very interesting technologies that are floating around. Many of them are coming from Clalit, which is the largest HMO in Israel. Half the country is covered by Clalit. They also own and operate 14 hospitals. Lots of innovation is coming out of the Clalit hospitals in terms of devices, new indications for old drugs, and a variety of different types of therapy."

"So, are you dealing with technology transfer and those issues?"

"It's definitely related. Some of the entities that we work with are tech transfer offices like Clalit has, in addition to all of the universities. Most of it is early stage."

"How would you describe some of the people you're working with?"

"Some of the inventors, a lot of the ones coming out of Clalit, have been working in whatever their specialty is, be it oncology or cardiology or whatever, for many, many years. And they have come up with inventions based on that clinical experience. We have also worked with some younger physicians and scientists who have come up with some ideas, generally more high-tech or telecom type projects. That might just be a function of the length of schooling and training you need to just get into the medical profession and then the number of years of experience that you need to have some kind of mastery in a field. So, the average age of the innovator is varied. In telecom and data security, it's full of people who came out of a unit in army intelligence called the 8200. And 8200 is almost like a factory for startups. If you're looking for an army connection there's a program in the army called the Atuda and it is a highly competitive academic track. And they have an engineering track, a medical track, and a number of other programs based on what the needs of the army are. They find the best of the brightest and they send them to college for Masters or PHDs or med school or whatever and then they serve in the army as officers working in their particular area," Schiffmiller said.

"So, it's kind of like here in the States where

somebody gets funded for med school or whatever and then they're obligated for a reciprocal amount of service for a certain amount of years."

"Exactly. And that is true for some of the programs coming out of the chief scientist office. It was always a matching type of thing, but they would fund programs with potential when even your uncle wouldn't give you money."

"I had an uncle like that. Was your background a mix of science and medicine or more in business?"

"I studied experimental psychology at Johns Hopkins a million years ago. Most of my career was a cross between technology and business. I don't have formal training as a scientist or in any of the life sciences but I've been working in the realm for more than 25 years so I've picked up what I need to know."

"In terms of innovation, what drives Israel? Jewish chutzpah?" I asked.

Dan Senor and Saul Singer, in the book Start-up Nation: The Story of Israel's Economic Miracle, describe how Israel's "adversity-driven culture, flattened hierarchies, and government policies create a society that uniquely combines both innovative and entrepreneurial intensity." The authors argue that, "Israel is not just a country, but a comprehensive state of mind. Where Americans emphasize decorum and exhaustive prep, Israelis put chutzpah over charm."

"I would not discount chutzpah. I think there is some reality around the fact that we're short on natural resources and none of our neighbors want to trade with us. I think in some cases we innovate because it's a culture that values improvisation. If you look at Israeli military history, we have had some great battles that were won by people who were on the ground, saw the problem, and took the initiative."

"Is all the influence based on innovation good?" I asked.

"I think that there's some influence for good and bad. On the one hand, Israeli companies are very innovative. On the other hand, a lot of them don't appear to aim to build a sustainable company. The aim is to come up with a great technology, commercialize it, as much as you need to, to have a big exit. I think part of it is this great nimble, improvisational mindset which is wonderful for coming up with the tech but it's not great for building a company that's going to be around for 50 years," Schiffmiller said.

"Any examples come to mind?" I asked.

"I was at a conference for startups probably about 10 years ago and one of the speakers was talking about raising money and everyone in the room was trying to raise money. And she was saying, well, you know, you can go to this kind of investor, you can go to that kind of investor. You can go public on the Tel Aviv Stock Exchange but that's not really considered an exit, that's just positioning you for your IPO on Nasdaq. And then she said, 'You can also raise money by selling more of your product.' And everyone started laughing."

CONCLUSION

As you hopefully have discovered, there are many key components in the success of Israel and Israeli medicine.

The military background, at times, sets the stage for lifelong friendships and business relationships. Many of the people I interviewed set up businesses with former military colleagues. Recruiters often take the best of the best from the military. And what has been invented in the military and proven to be medically viable is often carried over into the medical arena and used to establish new technology. A good example is the Pill Cam, derived from Popeye missile technology.

The Israeli culture itself is a key component, especially when it comes to joining forces with other countries and cultures. Singapore has a much more hierarchal and regimented business culture than Israel and consequently a less innovative milieu. The Israelis are a more irreverent, argumentative group. Certain cultural observers have stated that Jewish people really don't listen; instead they wait, and then make corrections after the other person speaks. But somehow the two cultures, Singapore and Israel, that would appear to be incompatible, come together in business ventures with truly remarkable outcomes.

Israeli culture allows an environment of creativity and enormous respect for education, with freedom to explore, fail, take risks, maybe fail again, roll with the punches, and hopefully someday succeed. How was all this created? Place in the middle of the desert tough people with the intoxicating desire to form a new nation ordained by the Torah. Take a mix of Russian immigration and incubators funded by the government and place them in a country fixated on survival and hungry for change. Add in the quintessential desire to ask questions, solve problems and improve the world and you have some of the formula for Israeli success. The rest of the ingredients, my dear readers, are a mix of faith, prayer, chutzpah, and magic, all ignited by certain mysterious, primordial forces that create a whole greater than the sum of its parts.

As with all countries and peoples, Israel has much room to grow and improve. The Israeli people endure

enormous ups and downs in a struggle to survive and
flourish in a tough neighborhood. I often use the example
of the Hillel sandwich for both a historical and modern
reference point. Hillel was a famous Jewish religious
leader and one of the most important figures in Jewish
history who is remembered during Passover. During the
Passover dinner, in the modern version, the Hillel
sandwich is eaten. It is usually composed of bitter herbs
such as horseradish (to remind us of the enslavement of
the Jewish nation in Egypt) and charoset (representative
of the mortar used by the Jewish slaves to build
storehouses in Egypt), a finely chopped sweet mixture of
fruits and nuts, typically apples, walnuts, red wine,
cinnamon, and honey) between two pieces of matzah
(cracker-like, unleavened bread that was eaten during the
times of fleeing from the wrath of Pharaoh when they
had to keep moving). Life in Israel today, like the Hillel
sandwich, is bitter-sweet.

Israel has made many mistakes. But I believe it is
always important to constructively critique and not
denigrate in order to improve the world. Of all the places
I have been, Israel, despite the tough exterior of its

people, is also among the most self-conscious about how it is seen in the eyes of the world. Part of this stems from delusional anti-Semitism and political prejudices. Perhaps one day the achievements of Israel will be judged, as it should be for all people, based on the actions and help it provides. So much needs to be done, and we can all work as a team to create life-enhancing and life-saving innovations. It seems much more productive to continue to put our efforts and energy into important fields such as medicine and technology that can change and improve lives instead of wasting billions of dollars on more wars and terrorism. Many of our individual frustrations, territorial aggressions, and violent destruction could diminish in the service of higher goals. The standard greeting in Israel, Shalom, means peace. And Israel clearly has created a world that will continue to provide new innovations and amazing gifts while promoting peace.

I hope you have enjoyed my book. Get ready for my next book on new advances in Israeli medicine, filled with refreshing new interviews and insights into The Start-Up Nation for Medical Innovation.

GENERAL REFERENCES

Chapter 2

Please view the following videos to learn about Doron Almog, his son Eran, and the Aleh Negev medical center and satellite clinics:

https://www.youtube.com/watch?v=9F6R2oQThXg&list=UUhm3sXHuDq1hJ1nCa2z_Dkw

https://www.youtube.com/user/alehisrael

https://www.youtube.com/watch?v=VEJSK3-kCTU

https://search.aol.com/aol/video?q=aleh+negev+israel&s_it=video-ans&sfVid=true&videoId=8446DDEA3255F595EA448446DDEA3255F595EA44&v_t=webmail-searchbox

https://www.youtube.com/watch?v=Ftnb2fpJ664 TEDx Tel Aviv

Special in Uniform. http://www.jpost.com/Israel-News/Politics-And-Diplomacy/Special-in-uniform-496192

Chapter 6

Cota D. The role of the endocannabinoid system in the regulation of hypothalamic-pituitary-adrenal axis activity. J Neuroendocrinol.;20 Suppl 1:35-8 (2008).

Correa F, Docagne F, Mestre L, et al. Cannabinoid system and neuroinflammation: implications for multiple sclerosis. Neuroimmunomodulation;14(3-4):182-187, (2007).

Correa F, Mestre L, Molina-Holgado E, et al. The role of cannabinoid system on immune modulation: therapeutic implications on CNS inflammation. Mini Rev Med Chem;5(7):671-675, (2005).

Gaoni Y and Mechoulam R. The structure and synthesis of cannabigerol, a new hashish constituent. Proc. Chem. Soc., 82 (1964).

Gaoni Yand Mechoulam R. Isolation, structure and partial synthesis of an active constituent of hashish. J. Amer. Chem. Soc., 86, 1646-1647 (1964).

Maccarrone M, Lorenzon T, Bari M, Melino G, Finazzi-Agrò A. Anandamide induces apoptosis in human cells via vanilloid receptors Evidence for a protective role of cannabinoid receptors. Journal of Biol Chem; 275 (41): 31938–31945, (2000).

Mechoulam R and Shvo Y. The structure of cannabidiol. Tetrahedron, 19, 2073-2078 (1963).

New Developments in Cannabinoid-Based Medicine: An Interview with Dr. Raphael Mechoulam in Longevity Medicine Review(http://www.lmreview.com/articles/view/new -developments-in-cannabinoid-based-medicine-an-interview-with-dr-raphael-mechoulam/)

Pagotto U, Marsicano G, Cota D, et al. The emerging role of the endocannabinoid system in endocrine regulation and energy balance. Endocr Rev;27(1):73-100, (2006).

Paher P and Kunos G. Modulating the endocannabinoid system in human health and disease: successes and failures. FEBS J; 280(9):1918-43, (2013).

Panikashvili D, Simeonidou C, Ben-Shabat S, et al. An endogenous cannabinoid (2-AG) is neuroprotective after brain injury. Nature;413(6855):527-531, (2001).

Pazos MR, Núñez E, Benito C, et al. Functional neuroanatomy of the endocannabinoid system. Pharmacol Biochem Behav;81(2):239-47, (2005).

Sparling PB, Giuffrida A, Piomelli D, et al. Exercise

activates the endocannabinoid system.
Neuroreport;14(17):2209-11, (2003).

http://healthland.time.com/2012/05/30/marijuana-
compound-treats-schizophrenia-with-few-side-effects-
clinical-trial/

https://www.israel21c.org/5-reasons-israel-is-
dominating-the-cannabis-industry/

https://www.israel21c.org/israel-to-become-major-
exporter-of-medical-cannabis/

https://www.israel21c.org/cannabis-extract-to-be-used-
to-treat-diabetes/

Chapter 7

Conan O'Brien visited Ziv during his tour of Israel.
Watch the video of Conan O'Brien visit to Israel and
the Ziv Hospital at
https://www.youtube.com/watch?v=khuUX79Qboo

Chapter 12

Nefesh B'Nefesh Media Coverage Sampling:

Times of Israel, July 19, 2016

Former marine, future soldiers fight nerves for journey 'home to Israel'.

http://www.timesofisrael.com/former-marine-future-soldiers-fight-nerves-for-journey-home-to-israel/

Yediot Achronot, July 26, 2016, Hebrew print edition and Ynet news

Summer of Love: US Jews come to Israel looking for a partner. www.ynetnews.com/articles/0,7340,L-4833689,00.html

Breitbart, July 21, 2016. Over 200 North American Immigrants Arrive in Israel.

http://www.breitbart.com/jerusalem/2016/07/21/watch-over-200-north-american-immigrants-arrive-in-israel/

Channel 2 News, Sivan Rahav-Meir, July 25, 2016. Dafna Meir obm, a nurse, was murdered at her door. Thousands of miles away, in the US, a young Jewish nurse, heard about this - and decided to do something:

http://www.jns.org/latest-articles/2016/8/3/israeli-nurse-to-israeli-nurse-a-love-story#.V6KNBJN97Uo=

https://www.facebook.com/NefeshBNefesh/posts/101
53806662192336

ABOUT THE AUTHOR

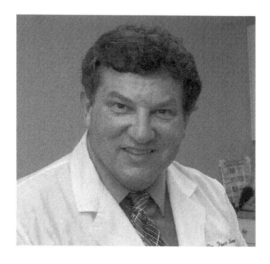

Dr. Robert A. Norman is a board-certified dermatologist and family practitioner who has been in practice for over 25 years. He is a faculty member for five medical schools (Clinical Professor) and has been honored with numerous service and teaching awards, including Physician of the Year (2005) and Distinguished Service Award (2007) in Hillsborough County, Tampa, Florida, Tampa Bay Medical Hero Award (2008), and the Hadassah Humanitarian Award (2012). Dr. Norman has written 40 books, including *The Blue Man and Other Stories of the Skin*, *Discover Magazine's Vital Signs--True Tales of Medical Mysteries, Obscure Diseases, and Life-Saving Diagnoses*, and *The Star of David*. He has been the editor and contributing writer of fifteen textbooks on Geriatrics and Geriatric Dermatology and published over 200 articles in various major media publications. He is the founding and current editor of the Springer Series on Clinical Cases in

Dermatology.

Dr. Norman has a private practice and is the chief physician and owner of Dermatology Healthcare, founded in 1994, which delivers essential skin care services for nursing home patients. He provides many national and international lectures each year; in October of 2007 he was the chairman and lecturer in Geriatric Dermatology at the World Congress of Dermatology in Buenos Aires, Argentina. In 2014 he was a Keynote Speaker at the Australasian Skin Cancer Conference in Brisbane, Australia, and was a co-chairman in Geriatric Dermatology at the World Congress of Dermatology in Vancouver in 2015. He spoke at the 2016 Pan-American Congress of Neurology and 40th Mexican Academy of Neurology Annual Meeting in 2016 on The Skin: Our Outer Brain. He also has both MPH and MBA degrees and was awarded the Doctor of Humane Letters after providing the commencement address at a major university.

He is a frequent medical volunteer and has participated in eight medical mission trips to serve the poor of southern Jamaica. Other trips have included Haiti, Cuba, and Guatemala. He is the current National Chairman of the Doctors for Israel for the Jewish National Fund.

To contact Dr. Norman for a lecture or speaking program based on this book or his other books, please email him at skindrrob@aol.com

20134283R00157

Made in the USA
Middletown, DE
09 December 2018